I0766834

Autophagy

Unlock the Secrets of Weight Loss, Anti-Aging, and Healing with Intermittent and Extended Water Fasting

Contents

Introduction

The following chapters will discuss everything that you need to know about the process of autophagy and how it can improve your daily life. Without the process of autophagy working properly in your body, dead and damaged cells and proteins start to build up. These parts get there through normal wear and tear on the body, but they need to be reduced to keep your body healthy. If they aren't removed and are instead allowed to just sit around, they can cause inflammation, along with a whole bunch of other health conditions.

The autophagic process is needed to ensure that your body can clear out these damaged and dead parts of cells effectively and timely. When this process is allowed to do its work, it can help reduce inflammation in the body, can make room for new cells throughout, and can prevent many other diseases.

One of the best ways to induce this process is to go on a fast. Whether you choose to try out intermittent fasting and some of the shorter-term fasts that come with it or if you want to go all-out and try an extended fast, you will find that fasting can put you into the autophagic process and get you the results, along with many others, that you are looking for. We will discuss how fasting can work with autophagy and why it is such a good idea.

For some people, fasting may not be the best choice. Due to medical and health conditions, they may not want to put themselves at risk through fasting. The good news is that there are other methods that you can choose, such as a protein fast, the ketogenic diet, and exercise, that will help you to get the same results without having to go for long periods without eating.

This guidebook details all of these topics and more. We will talk more about the benefits of autophagy, how to do a good fasting period to induce autophagy, the results that others have been able to get from this process, and even some tips that make fasting easier to start on and stick with in the long run. There is so much to learn about and understand when it comes to the autophagic process – and this guidebook aims to help with it all.

When you are ready to improve your health, reduce your risks of inflammation and other diseases, fight off cancer, and even lose weight, then make sure to check out this guidebook and learn more about the autophagic process.

Chapter 1: The What and the Why – What Really Is Autophagy, and Why Are People Interested in It?

Even if your body is healthy and you aren't suffering from any illnesses, diseases, or pain, cells are constantly being damaged as part of a normal and healthy metabolic process. This occurs just by living our daily lives – and it is not a big deal. As we age, deal with more stress, and have more and more free radical damage throughout the body, the cells start to increase their rate of being damaged more than ever.

This is where the process of autophagy comes into play. This is the natural process in the body that helps clear up damaged cells inside and includes cells that have gotten old and do not serve any functional purposes but haven't been removed out of organs and tissues yet. While it is natural for the body to get old and have damaged cells, it is not a good idea to have them stay around. You need to remove these cells because they can trigger inflammatory pathways and will end up contributing to a wide range of diseases as well.

The word 'autophagy' was coined more than forty years ago. It comes from the Greek words *auto*, which means self, and *phagy*, which means eating. Hence, basically, the body is going to be the process of self-eating. This may not sound like the best thing in the world; however, it is a natural and completely good thing to occur in your body. What this means is that the body is going to clean itself out, removing all the old and damaged cells, to allow more room for the healthy cells that you want to have there.

It has only been in the past few years that researchers have actually had a chance to observe the process of autophagy. What they have found is that autophagy can help promote longevity and provides a ton of benefits when it comes to your metabolism, heart, immune system, and nervous system. Let's take a more in-depth look at the process of autophagy and why it is such a great thing to implement into your own daily routine.

What Is Autophagy?

The first thing that we need to take a look at is the process of autophagy. The definition of autophagy is the consumption of the body's own tissues as a metabolic process occurring in starvation and in certain diseases – this is just a convoluted sentence which means that the body will use its own processes to eat up and remove tissues in the body. This process usually happens during fasting and when certain diseases occur. Researchers think that this is a type of survival mechanism or a way that the body can respond to stress in your life to keep itself protected.

The next thing to look at is whether autophagy is a bad thing or a good thing for your health. Autophagy is a *very* good thing for your life. As touched on earlier, autophagy is "self-eating of the body," which may sound a bit strange, but it is a completely healthy and normal way for the body to go through the cellular renewal process. In fact, autophagy is going to be so beneficial that it is seen as one of the biggest keys to preventing many common diseases, such as diabetes, cancer, liver disease, infections, and autoimmune diseases.

One of the first benefits that you will notice with autophagy is that it can help prevent many of the causes linked to aging. The reason that it is so successful with this is that it helps destroy and then reuse any damaged components that are likely to occur in the spaces within the cells. What this means is that autophagy is going to work by using the waste that the cells produce in order to create brand-new materials that are used for building up and repairing different parts of the body.

There are not many long-term studies about autophagy, but from some of the ones that have recently come out, we know that autophagy is important to clean up the body and defend against some of the negative effects that bother us due to stress in our modern world. However, the way that this works is something that is not completely understood yet, which could make it hard to understand why this is a process that is so necessary and beneficial. However, as more research is done, we will be able to learn more about the whole process and put it to more use for our needs.

A few different steps are involved when it comes to the autophagic process. First, lysosomes are the part of the cells that will go in and destroy large damaged structures, such as the mitochondria of the cells, and then take those damaged parts out of the cell, using them as a form of fuel. When the damaged cells are used as fuel, they can then be eliminated out of the body just like any other type of waste.

Without this autophagic process occurring, some issues can arise. The damaged and old cells and parts are just going to stick around the body, and they will never be able to clean themselves up. This makes it hard for the cells, and the parts they make up, to heal themselves. This can lead to inflammation, chronic diseases, and more.

How Was Autophagy Discovered?

Keith R. Porter and his student Thomas Ashford from the Rockefeller Institute were some of the first to observe the autophagic process. In January of 1962, they reported that they saw a higher number of lysosomes in rat liver cells after they added in glucagon to the diet and that some of these displaced lysosomes found near the center of the rat cells were holding onto other cell organelles like the mitochondria.

They called this process autolysis. However, Porter and Ashford were wrong about their interpretation of the data. They assumed that this was a part of lysosome formation. However, lysosomes can't be organelles in the cells since they are part of the cytoplasm, and the hydrolytic enzymes are going to be produced by the microbodies.

It was then in 1963 that Hruban, Spargo, and their colleagues were able to publish a very detailed description of what they were able to call 'focal cytoplasmic degradation'. This study was able to reference a study that was done in Germany in 1955 that looked at injury induced sequestration. This study recognized that there were three stages of maturation of the sequestered cytoplasm to lysosomes and that this process was not something that had to be limited to the body being injured. This was then the first time that the lysosomes of the cells were established as the main site and source of the autophagic process.

It wasn't until the 1990s, though, that a new era of research into autophagy began to take hold. During this time, there was more than one group of researchers whom all discovered genes that were related to autophagy using budding yeast, and all of these groups were able to do so independently. And then, in 2003, a unified nomenclature was advocated to list out the autophagy genes that had been discovered.

In 1999, there was a landmark discovery that linked autophagy and cancer. And, to date, this is still a major theme when it comes to researching autophagy. The roles of autophagy in immune defense and other neurological disorders have seen much attention over the years as well.

The idea of autophagy has definitely seen many changes throughout the years. While there is still much research that needs to be done concerning this topic and how it can benefit humans, there has already been a lot of interest in this topic throughout the world. Research that began over forty years ago is now being used to see how well autophagy can help with a bunch of different diseases and conditions of the body, and being able to work with this process and figure out how to induce this process, can ensure you prevent and keep away many different diseases of the body.

The Benefits of Autophagy

This chapter has discussed a bit about autophagy, but there are so many other benefits that come with the process. It is time to talk about them now. Some of the research that has been done concerning autophagy suggests that some of the benefits that you will find when you encourage this process include:

- Provides the cells with the energy and the building blocks that they need on a molecular level.
- Recycles all the damaged parts of the cells, including the organelles, proteins, and aggregates.
- Helps the mitochondria to regulate their own functions. When this happens, the cell can produce more energy and won't have to deal with as much damage from oxidative stress.
- Clears out the peroxisomes and the endoplasmic reticulum when they are damaged.
- Protects the nervous system better than anything else. It can also help by encouraging the nerve cells of the brain to grow more. Because of this, and other factors, it seems that autophagy can improve cognitive function, neuroplasticity, and brain structure.
- It helps support the growth of the cells in the heart and can protect against many diseases of the heart.

• Enhances the immune system to keep us feeling strong and healthy. It does this by getting rid of many pathogens that show up in the body.

• Defends against the misfolded and toxic proteins that will contribute to a variety of different diseases through the body.

• Can ensure that the stability of your DNA is protected. When DNA is damaged, it can make the genes behave in a way that is not natural. This can make you more predisposed to a variety of conditions that can be hard to deal with.

• Can prevent any unnecessary damage to the healthy organs and tissues of the body so they can continue with their own process.

• Can potentially help with a wide variety of other issues, including fighting cancer and dealing with neurodegenerative diseases. There still needs to be more research done to determine how and if autophagy can help fight cancer, but so far, the research looks promising, and this may be exactly what we need to help deal with the horrible disease.

There are also a few different types of autophagy that you may come across in your studies. Macroautophagy is the one that is talked about in this guidebook and is the most common. This type of autophagy is going to be known as an "evolutionarily conserved catabolic process involving the formation of vesicles that engulf the cellular macromolecules and organelles." To make it simple, this kind is basically the one that will find the damaged and old cells in the body, and then clean them all out so that the body will perform the way that you want it to.

What is interesting here is that humans are not the only species who can benefit from the process of autophagy. There are many other organisms too that will see this process happen, including mammals, flies, plants, mold, worms, and yeast. Most of the research that is out there about autophagy has been done with rats and yeast, but more and more studies are now being done to see how autophagy will affect humans and all of the great benefits that can come with this process in your life.

Is There a Relationship Between Autophagy and Apoptosis?

First, we need to understand what apoptosis is. Apoptosis is the death of cells that occurs as a normal and controlled part of the organism's growth or development. Researchers looking at autophagy believe that this process is going to be selective about what it is going to remove out of the body. There is not any clear evidence that either autophagy or apoptosis controls the other process, but some beginning studies do indicate that autophagy is a mechanism of apoptosis independent cell death.

One main reason that there is such an interest in this kind of relationship is that many researchers now believe that autophagy may be a process that, when used properly, could help treat many neurodegenerative diseases, and cancer, thanks to the ability of the process to modulate cell death. It is possible that autophagy can act kind of like a therapeutic target, ensuring that the harmful materials are removed, and protecting any cells that are considered healthy.

While there needs to be more research done to see how true this is and what can be done to make it more effective, it is possible that, in the future, we could use autophagy to protect all of the healthy cells that we do not want to die, and destroy and remove all of the cells that are damaged or diseased.

How Can I Induce Autophagy?

The third question that we need to ask at this point is how you can induce this process of autophagy. We already know that there are a ton of benefits of choosing this kind of process, and now you are probably wondering what you need to do to induce this process and see amazing results.

Autophagy is active in all cells, but it is going to be increased in response to stress or some kind of nutrient deprivation, such as starvation or fasting. This means that you can choose to work with good stressors in the form of exercise or with a temporary calorie restriction, such as fasting, to boost the autophagic processes. Both of these strategies have been linked to many good benefits, such as longevity, weight control, and the inhibition of many diseases that are associated with aging.

Let's take a look at some of the different methods that we can use to induce autophagy in your own life.

Practice fasting

When it comes to some of the lifestyle and diet habits that you can control, the thing that you can do that will trigger autophagy is fasting. You can even use the common dietary strategy that is called intermittent fasting. Fasting is a very simple concept. You will increase your fasting window while decreasing your eating window. You would still have a lot of liquids and waters, as long as they don't have any calories in them, to keep your body hydrated and help you get through the fast.

If you don't know about intermittent fasting, we will take a look at it a bit later on in more detail. However, intermittent fasting is cyclical fasting that will involve time-restricted eating. There are many different types of intermittent fasting, and all of them will be pretty effective – you just need to decide the method that works the best for you.

Now, you may be wondering how long you need to go on a fast for in order to achieve autophagy? Studies suggest that you should go on a fast that is between one to two days long to get the most benefits. However, this is a long time, and it isn't always the easiest for people to do. It is best to aim for at least a sixteen-hour fast in the beginning and see if you can build up from there. Even these shorter fasts can promote autophagy throughout the body.

An easy way to do one of these smaller fasts is to stick with just one or two meals a day, rather than three meals and a bunch of snacks. If you do end up finishing your dinner at about seven o'clock at night, then try not eating anything until eleven o'clock or noon the next day, and skipping breakfast in the process. This allows you to be on a fast that promotes autophagy, without feeling deprived in the process.

You can also choose to go on an occasional fast that lasts two to three days once you have time to gain more experience with fasting. If you do find that alternate day fasting works for you, then you need to restrict your calorie amount during the fasting days to either nothing, or do a variation that allows for 500 calories. Then, on the days that you are not fasting, make sure that you eat a healthy and nutritious diet to help support autophagy even more.

Fasting of all kinds can help you see results when you are trying to induce autophagy. You can choose to go on an extended water fast, which will take about seven to ten days, of only drinking water and avoiding food. Sometimes this may seem like a stretch for going on the fast, and most people will choose to only go on an intermittent fast – one that usually lasts for less than 36 hours overall. However, you can choose the type of fasting that most interests you, and then implement that into your own schedule in order to see the autophagic process show up in your life.

Think about going on the ketogenic diet

Another method that you can try to use to help promote the process of autophagy in your life is to consider going on the ketogenic diet. The ketogenic diet is a diet that is very low carb and very high fat and provides some of the same results in the body as fasting – without any fasting or longer periods of not eating. The keto diet is going to involve getting around 75 percent of your calories from fat each day, and no more than five percent of your calories out of carbs. The rest can come from moderate amounts of protein.

The reason that you would want to go with this kind of diet plan is because it changes up the metabolism in the body, forcing you to stop using the readily available glucose (which is almost gone now that you are limiting your intake so much), and has the body rely on healthy fats for fuel instead. This can help you to speed up the metabolism, burn the extra fat and weight hanging around the body, and make you feel better.

What are some of the most beneficial foods to use when you want to follow the ketogenic diet? You will want to go with foods that are whole and high in fat, such as nuts and seeds, avocado, fermented cheeses, grass-fed meat, ghee, butter, eggs, olive oil, and higher-fat choices of meat. Vegetables can be included, especially the ones that have a lot of fiber in them – as long as you keep the carb content in them as low as possible.

In response to limiting your carbs so much, you will see ketone bodies formed, and these are going to have many effects that protect various organs and tissues. Some studies suggest that this process of ketosis is also going to cause starvation-induced autophagy, which can help the body out in so many different ways.

For example, in one animal study that was done, rats were put on the ketogenic diet. In this study, the keto diet was able to start the autophagic pathways that reduced brain injury, both during and after seizures. This is definitely an area that is going to need more time and research in the future, but it can show just how great the ketogenic diet can be when you want to get the process of autophagy started in your body.

Exercise

Another one of the good stressors that you need to worry about when you want to start the autophagic process is exercise. Recent research shows how exercise can help to induce this process in several organs, especially the ones that are the most involved in regulating the metabolism, such as the adipose tissue, pancreas, liver, and muscles.

While many benefits come with exercise, it can be considered a form of stress because it will break down tissue throughout the body. These tissues need to be repaired so that they can grow back stronger than ever. Right now, studies are uncertain about how much exercise you will need to do in order to start or boost up autophagy. However, it is suggested that doing intense exercise can be the most beneficial to help you see these kinds of results.

When you are working on the muscle tissue that is cardiac and skeletal, you could find that just 30 minutes of exercise could be enough to induce autophagy. In addition, you could exercise while you are in one of the fasts as well, which helps you get even better results in the process.

Some Precautions to Consider About Autophagy and Fasting

There is still a lot that researchers need to find out concerning autophagy and how best to induce it or even boost it. Beginning to induce autophagy by incorporating fasting and regular exercise into your routine is often a fantastic place to start. Both of these things, especially when they are combined together, can provide the body with many benefits in addition to autophagy.

However, if you are on certain medications that are meant to help control different health conditions, it may be a good idea to talk to your doctor before you decide to get started on a fasting regiment. People who suffer from diabetes or hypoglycemia, and women who are either pregnant or breastfeeding, should never fast. Anyone who is dealing with or being treated for a disease, such as cancer, should make sure that they discuss this option with their doctor before starting as well.

There are so many great benefits to enjoy when it comes to the process of autophagy. This is a simple process that can really make a difference in your overall health and can stop many common diseases that seem to take over as we age and make us sick. Finding ways to induce or boost this process, such as through fasting, trying out diets like the ketogenic diet, or exercising, can ensure that the body cleans itself out and feels the very best.

Chapter 2: How Does It Work – The Science Behind What Happens to Our Bodies When We Fast

As mentioned in the previous chapter, fasting can be one of the main ways that you can enter the autophagic process, and it can be a great way to boost this process as well. Fasting allows the body to enter into a starvation mode for a bit, which can signal to the body that it is time to clean itself out of all the damaged and old parts and use them as fuel instead of relying on the food that we are used to enjoying.

The next question here is – what actually happens to our bodies when we go on a fast. Why is the process of autophagy so prevalent and work so efficiently to clear out the body, by only skipping a few meals along the way? Let's take a look at some of the things that will happen to your body when you decide to add fasting to your life and why it is so effective at helping you to start the process of autophagy.

About four or five hours after you are done eating, you will notice that the levels of insulin in your body are going to start falling. When these levels fall, this will trigger a series of hormonal changes because we start to enter into the fasting state. The first step here is that the body will use any readily accessible stores of glucose, or glycogen, to keep the body going and provide us with energy. After about ten to twelve hours, these stores are going to be depleted, and the body will begin to look for another source of fuel to keep it going. From there, the body will start to rely on stored fat in the body to keep itself going and full of energy.

The switch from glucose to fat as the biggest source of fuel in the body is key for many health benefits that come with fasting. It is going to take about twelve hours after your last meal before the body can use up all of the glucose stores that it has, and before it will start to use fat for energy. This is why you want to consider going on a 24-hour or longer fast. This ensures that you get at least twelve hours of fat burning out of the process. Of course, the amount of energy that you are going to derive from the excess stored body fat can vary between each person, and some of the things that it will depend on include:

- Whether you are metabolically flexible or fat adapted – what this means is whether your body is adapted to switching over to fat burning or not.

- How much glycogen is stored in the body – this will often depend on how many carbs you have eaten in your meals, and how much glycogen the muscles and liver can hold onto as well.

- How quickly you can deplete those glycogen sores – this is often going to depend on how active you can be during these fasting periods.

- Once the insulin levels throughout the body have had enough time to fall efficiently so that fat will start to release out of its stores, then your body can burn fat instead of glucose, and you can start to reap some of the benefits in the process.

How Will My Body Change When I Am on a Fast?

Now that we have taken some time to look at what fasting can do, and how important it is for the body to start relying on the stored body fat to get more energy, it is time to take a look at some of the ways that our bodies are going to change when we fast on a regular basis. You will be amazed at some of the dramatic changes that can happen in the body as the fasting time progresses. Some of the most dramatic changes include:

- The levels of blood glucose are going to fall, which means that the levels of insulin will decrease as well. The cells are going to detect that there is a decrease in these levels. This forces them to stop being in a growth phase, and they will enter into the repair phase.
- Blood glucose levels are going to be stopped from falling too low too quickly thanks to the liver. When these blood glucose levels start to go down, the liver is going to work to increase its own glucose production.
- As the levels of insulin continue to decrease, the cells are going to develop a bigger sensitivity to the effects of insulin. This means that over time, and with the right fasting method, it is possible that the individual could see a decrease in their insulin resistance and an improvement in their glucose tolerance test results.
- In addition, the decreases in both the blood glucose and insulin levels are going to be even bigger in those individuals who are dealing with diabetes when they get started.
- You will also see that the secretion of glucagon during this time is further going to encourage the fat burning that you want with fasting.

- The biggest changes in insulin and with fat burning are often going to occur sometime between eighteen and 24 hours of fasting. This is why the longer fast can sometimes be a better option since the benefits are going to multiply themselves.

- As the fasting time progresses, the liver will then start to produce ketones from stored body fat to provide us with fuel. As the ketone level starts to rise in the blood, the brain can take up these ketones for its own energy.

- Leptin levels are going to start to fall, reaching their greatest decline after 36 hours. This may mean that you feel more hungry during the first day to a day and a half on the fast, but then it may go down a bit.

- Another thing to notice is that the hormone activity of the thyroid is going to increase at first. Then after 24 to 36 hours, it is going to decrease. This is going to be accompanied by an initial increase in the rate of the metabolism, and then there will be a nice gradual decrease.

- Those who go on a fast will also notice that their total cholesterol and the HDL or high-density lipoprotein will rise during the fast. This is because fat is now being transported around the body as fuel and is not a big deal.

- The growth hormone production is going to head up during this time, which is a good way to encourage fat burning while also protecting the muscles, so they aren't broken down for glucose.

- You will see that the insulin-like growth factor levels will start to see a decrease as well.

- There will be some changes in the brain which are going to produce chemicals that enhance nerve growth and can bring about a sense of well-being.

These are all changes that you can see in your body when you decide to go on a fast. The longer fasts are more likely to see more of these benefits than others because the body has more time to show off these benefits. However, some changes are not going to happen as quickly or necessarily to the extent in those who are metabolically inflexible or those who are obese compared to those who have more tolerance and are more used to fasting, or those who are lean. It could take a few fasts in some individuals before these changes are instigated into your life smoothly.

As the body has some time to adapt to the fast, there are going to be a ton of benefits that come with it. We will talk about these in a bit, but you will see that a good fast can: reduce fat in the body, reduce the issues that can come with insulin resistance, which in turn decreases the risk of heart disease and diabetes, as well as a reduction in inflammation and disorders that come with these, and even the inhibition of cell growth, especially in cells that could be cancerous.

The Health Benefits of Fasting

When it comes to going on a fast, many different benefits can come with being on one. Many people don't realize the benefits that come with just a short fast, much less the number of benefits you will get if you decide to go on a longer fast. Let's take a look at some of the health benefits of fasting, and why it can be one of the best ways to see the changes that occur in your body thanks to fasting.

Can change the way that the hormones and cells function

When you spend more time not eating, there are a few different things that can happen to your body. To start, the body can initiate important cellular repair processes (namely the process of autophagy), and it can change up the hormone levels to ensure that stored body fat is easier to get to. There are a number of changes that will show up in your body while you are fasting that relate to this topic, and they include:

- Gene expression: There are going to be some changes in your molecules and genes when you go on a fast, especially the ones that are responsible for protecting you against diseases and helping you to live longer.
- Cellular repair: The body is going to induce many different repair processes on a cellular level when you are on a fast. This can include removing any material that is considered waste from the cells.
- Human growth levels: The levels of growth hormone found in the blood could increase by five times when you are fasting. These higher levels of the growth hormone help with a gain in muscle and fat burning, as well as providing you with many other benefits.
- Insulin levels: You will find that on a fast, the levels of insulin in the blood can drop quite a bit, which will facilitate fat burning.

You will see weight loss

One of the benefits of autophagy, as well as fasting, is weight loss. Unless you spend a lot of time overcompensating for the amount of time that you weren't eating, it is possible that you will lose some weight. There are a number of reasons for this. For example, having lower levels of insulin and higher levels of growth hormone can help you break down fat in the body easier, and you can use this as energy. Because of this, short-term fasting can increase your metabolism by up to fourteen percent, making it easier to burn even more calories than before.

Fasting can work on both sides of this calorie equation. You will find that it will boost your metabolic rate, which means that it increases the number of calories that go out. Fasting can also do wonders by reducing how much food you eat during your eating times, unless you go crazy, which can reduce the calories that you take in.

Can reduce inflammation and oxidative stress throughout the body

As many studies are showing, oxidative stress is actually one of the main steps towards chronic diseases and aging. What happens with this is that unstable molecules, which go by the name of free radicals, get into the body. These free radicals are not supposed to be there, and they are very good at reacting with some of the other important molecules, like your DNA and protein, and causing much damage to them.

There are numerous studies out there that show how intermittent fasting can actually help the body become more resistant to this oxidative stress. In addition to this, fasting can help fight off inflammation, which is another problem for many common diseases that are associated with aging and a poor diet.

Can help keep your heart health

Heart disease is considered one of the biggest killers throughout the world. And because there are so many risk factors out there that can cause heart disease, it is no wonder that we need to always be on the lookout to ensure our hearts stay as strong and healthy as possible.

It is commonly known that there are different risk factors or health markers that are associated with either an increase or a decrease in your risk of developing heart disease. Fasting is known to help improve several of the risk factors. Some of the ways that fasting can help is by lowering blood pressure and helping with blood sugar levels, blood triglycerides, LDL cholesterol, and inflammatory markers.

This one will need to have a bit more research done on it before we can know for sure. A lot of the information about how effective fasting can be on our heart health is based on animal studies. However, it stands to reason that if you stick with the protocols that come with your fasting method, you will increase the metabolism and burn off more of that excess body fat, which is seen as one of the biggest risk factors to heart disease. Add in a healthy diet when you do eat, and you will see a big difference in your health.

Can help with a variety of repair processes in the cells

When we fast, the cells that are inside the body are going to start the autophagic process in order to get rid of all the wastes in the cells. This is going to involve the cells getting broken down and then being metabolized. This ensures that all of these old and damaged parts of the cells are broken down and then sent out of the body to keep you healthier. Increasing the autophagy that occurs in the body may protect against many different types of disease, such as cancer and Alzheimer's.

You can see changes in your brain health

Anything that provides many benefits to the body will also provide many benefits to the brain. Fasting has been known to improve a lot of other features of the metabolism that are also important for the health of your brain. This could include a reduction in oxidative stress, a reduction in the amount of inflammation in the body, and even a reduction in the resistance to insulin and blood sugar levels.

There have been different studies done that show how intermittent fasting may increase the growth of new nerve cells, which is going to have a ton of benefits for how well the brain can function. It is also going to increase the number of BDNF (brain-derived neurotrophic factor). When there is a deficiency of this, it could be a cause of depression and other problems of the brain.

Can help extend your lifespan and help you live longer than before

One of the best parts of being on a fast is that it can help extend your lifespan if you follow it properly. There have been several studies done that show how fasting in all forms can extend your lifespan in a similar way to what has been seen with continuous calorie restriction. In addition, some of these studies showed that the effects of the fast were very dramatic. In fact, one of these studies showed that the rats who went on a fast every alternate day were able to live up to 83 percent longer compared to the rats who didn't fast at all.

While more studies still need to be done on this (it is hard to measure longevity in humans because of how long they live to start with), fasting is definitely something that has become popular among those who favor anti-aging. And given the fact that there are many metabolic benefits of fasting, and all of the benefits of other health markers with fasting, it does make sense that this could be the right tool to help you live a healthier, and longer, life.

There are so many benefits that come with going on a fast. It can help the body to remove much of the waste that it has inside. It can help us to feel younger and can prevent aging. And it even helps with weight loss, the functioning of the brain, and so much more. When it comes to implementing the process of autophagy, something that is very much a part of all these things, fasting is one of the best methods to use to see a ton of results.

Special Considerations for Women Who Want to Use Fasting

Now that we have introduced the idea of fasting, it is time to look specifically on how fasting can work for women. It is important that women understand that they need to handle the fast a bit differently than men. Some women can go on any of the fasting protocols we list here, and they won't have any problems at all. However, others may find that fasting is too extreme, or they need to take it slowly to see how their bodies react, rather than jumping right in.

Many women do experience some issues when it comes to fasting. They can see their metabolism slow down, issues with their reproductive system, fewer or no periods, and even early menopause. This is why it is so important for women to take some extra precautions when they want to go on any type of fast for their health.

To keep this simple, it seems that going on a fast, especially some of the longer-term fasts, can cause a hormonal imbalance for some women, especially if they are not careful and they don't go on the fast properly. Women and their hormones seem to be extremely sensitive, at least more so than men, to any signals of starvation in the environment. If the body feels as if it is being starved, it is going to start ramping up its own production of ghrelin and leptin, which are the hunger hormones in the body.

So, when women go on a fast and start to feel overly hungry after they under-eat, they are experiencing this process happening. Their hormones are increasing, and this causes them to be hungry – this is basically the female body trying to protect a potential fetus, even if you are not pregnant or have no plans to become pregnant in the near future.

When you continue on the fast and try to ignore these intense hunger cues, it just makes them worse. Often we fail and binge later on, before following all of that up with some more undereating and starvation again in the hopes that we can finally get it right. It is this vicious cycle that throws the hormones out of control, and if care is not taken, it may cause the halt to ovulation in some women.

In some animal studies that have been done, after two weeks of an intermittent fast, the female rats stopped having their menstrual cycles, and there was shrinkage in the ovaries. In addition, these female rats experienced more insomnia compared to their male counterparts. The men did suffer a little with lower testosterone production while fasting but did not see as dramatic effects as women.

Right now, there are not as many human studies that have been done to look at the differences between how women and men do on these kinds of fasts, but if the animal studies we look at can confirm anything, it is that going on this kind of fasting for too long could throw off the hormonal balance in some women. This could cause issues like fertility problems and may make various eating disorders like binge eating, bulimia, and anorexia more prevalent as well.

If you don't go on a fast properly, it can be hard on the body, especially if you are new to the whole idea, or you jump into it without proper preparation. So, if you are a woman and it is your first time doing any fast, you may find that doing a modified version of fasting, or a crescendo fasting, will work the best for you. This helps the body ease into the fasting regimen, which can make it easier for the body to adjust without feeling like it is going into starvation.

With crescendo fasting, you only need to do a fast a few days each week, rather than trying to do it every day. This is a great way for you to get the benefits of fasting without accidentally throwing your hormones out of place. If you find that you can do this kind of fasting without any issues, then you can increase the amount of time, or the number of days, that you go on a fast. This method is easier and gentler and helps the body adapt better to the fasting regimen without problems.

Not all women are going to need to start with a crescendo fasting, but it can definitely be a good option to go with. It ensures that you are going to see success, and gently eases the body into the fasting regimen without having anything be overdone in the process.

Now, the rules that come with crescendo fasting are pretty easy to follow, and you will find that the fasting periods aren't as long and you still feel some of the benefits that come with it. Some of the rules that you should follow when it comes to crescendo fasting include:

> 1. Pick out two or three nonconsecutive days during the week that you will go on a fast. You may choose to do Tuesday, Thursday, and Saturday if you want to work with three days, for example.

2. On the fasting days, you can do a bit of exercise, but make sure it is something simple and not too strenuous. Try out a nice walk around the block or some yoga.

3. For these fasts, you do not want to go for a long period of time. Twelve to sixteen hours is usually enough to get the results you want and ease your body into the process of fasting.

4. On the other days of the week, eat normal and healthy diets. You can also do HIIT (high-intensity interval training) or strength training on these days to help keep you active.

5. Make sure that you drink plenty of water, especially during the fasting period. It is fine to have some coffee or tea on occasion to mix things up, just don't add in any sweetener or milk.

6. After two to three weeks, evaluate how you are feeling. If you feel that things are going well and you can handle more, go ahead and add in another day of fasting to your week.

7. An optional thing that you can try out when you go on this crescendo fasting is to take about five to eight grams of BCAAs during the fast. These are known as branched chain amino acids and taking this supplement does have a few calories, but not enough to throw you off your fast. This is going to provide some extra fuel to your muscles so you can stay strong while fasting, and it helps to take the edge off fatigue and hunger.

Going on the crescendo fast is not something that everyone has to do. And if you feel that another form of fasting is better for you, then go ahead and try it out. There is no one-size-fits-all when it comes to the world of fasting and seeing results from autophagy, which is why there are so many protocols that you can choose from.

However, because some women are very sensitive to changes in food and the environment, it is not always best to jump right into fasting. This can mess with the system and make it hard to keep things in line. Working with an easier fast, such as the crescendo fast, can ensure that you get the benefits of this fast, without having to worry about the negative side effects that could come from your hormones getting messed up.

Everyone can benefit from a little fasting in their lives. Whether you decide to go all out and try to work alternate day fasting or you want to ease into it with one of the other methods we will talk about you will find that there are a ton of benefits that come with this eating strategy.

Chapter 3: Myths vs. Truths – Common Misconceptions About Autophagy and Fasting

Before we get into more information about fasting and what it all entails, it is important to dispel some of the common myths and misconceptions that can come with the idea of fasting and autophagy. These misconceptions are going to make it hard to convince some people that going on a fast is actually a good idea. We have spent years hearing about how we need to eat every few hours and that skipping meals is such a bad thing for us – when, in reality, it can help to speed up our metabolisms and the process of autophagy.

Let's take a look at some of the most common myths that are out there about fasting and autophagy and come to understand why they are instead really good for our overall health.

Fasting Is Going to Put Your Body in Starvation Mode

One common misconception that many people will have when it comes to going on a fast is that fasting will put you into starvation mode. Starvation mode is the period in your body where the metabolism shuts down to conserve energy because you have gone a long time without food. If starvation mode occurs too much, it can mess with the metabolism and make weight loss almost impossible.

However, for the most part, unless you do something really off with your fast, you will see some amazing benefits when you go on a fast, without ever having to worry about going into starvation mode at the same time. Most research shows that it takes at least 72 hours before starvation mode becomes a big problem for most people. Since many people decide that they will stick with intermittent fasting, they will be on and off the fast before these issues even come up.

Even if you do go on a longer fast, as long as you aren't fasting all of the time, and you eat a healthy diet beforehand, you don't have to worry about starvation mode. Starvation mode is only going to be an issue when the individual decides to go on a fast for a very long time, or they go too extreme with their fasting rules. For example, if you go on a two-week fast every month and then cut your calories down to 800 for the rest of the month, you are probably not giving the body the nutrients it needs. If you go on a twenty-hour fast each day, and then only eat 500 calories after that, then there are issues as well.

The most important thing to remember about starvation mode is that the body needs to feel that it is really short on nutrients and that it is likely not to get those nutrients soon. It goes into this mode as a way to deal with the lack of nutrients. If you keep your fasts reasonable, and make sure that you take in enough calories each day, or overall, with healthy and nutritious foods, then you can enjoy going on a fast and experiencing the autophagic process, without having to worry about starvation mode.

Fasting Is Going to Make You Overeat and Can Ruin the Effects of Autophagy

One common concern that comes up when we talk about fasting and autophagy is the idea that once you are done with the fast, you are going to overeat, and then all of the benefits will be canceled out. It is true that you are going to be incredibly hungry when you are done with fasting; however, this doesn't mean that you have to give in to those cravings and those urges along the way.

This is where some planning needs to come in. You may have the best resolution in the world to not overeat and to stay healthy and get all of the benefits from fasting, but then you go some time without eating, and you get hungry. When your eating window finally opens again, you are going to be really hungry, and your body will crave everything sweet and unhealthy. Without some planning, it is possible that you will end up overeating.

This doesn't mean that you are counteracting all the benefits of the autophagy that occurred during that time. However, it is something that you need to work on a bit. Meal planning can definitely be the answer that you are looking for if you decide to go on a fast to help with weight loss as well.

When you come up with a meal plan, consider adding a few extra calories into the beginning meal, or the first one that you have after you finish the fast. And perhaps consider having a healthier "treat" on there. In the beginning, you are going to have cravings, and they will be hard to deal with. And you are going to be hungry. Don't ignore this. Rather than trying to split up the calories completely evenly when you have three meals after the fast, give the first meal some extra calories, and cut the others down a little bit. This helps you to eat a little extra and satisfy those cravings, while also ensuring that you aren't going to feel deprived.

Fasting Is Bad for Your Health

If you read the previous chapter, you know that it is not true that fasting is bad for your health. We have had some long-held beliefs that fasting is a horrible thing for our bodies. We assume that it is going to put our bodies into starvation mode, that we are going to feel miserable, and that we will have such a slow metabolism from missing even one meal that we can kiss losing weight goodbye forever.

But does any of this really make sense? Does it make sense that we would enter starvation mode just from missing a meal or two? Our ancestors didn't have a ton of food just sitting around, and they may have had to go several days without getting any good at all. Does this mean that they went into starvation mode and their metabolisms were ruined all the time?

Have you ever been sick and had to go a few days without eating? Whether you were just suffering from the flu and didn't have anything to eat for a few days, or you were throwing up and couldn't keep anything down, we have all gone without eating during that time as well. Did that mean we entered into starvation mode and our metabolisms were ruined forever?

Of course not. Our bodies are designed to take a little bit of stress, and missing a meal here or there is not a big deal. Studies and research have shown that you can go up to 72 hours on a fast before the big side effects of starvation mode start to become an issue. And as long as you make sure that your diet is full of healthy and nutritious foods when you are no longer fasting, it is easy to add in the daily, or a few times a week, fasts that are common with intermittent fasting.

If you can add one of the protocols of fasting into your routine, you are going to get a whole host of benefits out of the process. You will get to enjoy a healthier heart, weight loss, mental clarity, better blood pressure, fewer issues with insulin resistance and diabetes, and so much more – all it takes it putting the body on a short fast on occasion and allowing the process of autophagy to take control.

Fasting and Autophagy Will Burn Off Muscles

Studies that take a look at alternate daily fasting show that the concern over losing muscle on a fast is misplaced. Alternate daily fasting over a period that was 70 days long did see a decrease in body weight of an average of six percent in participants. However, the fat mass of those same individuals did increase by eleven point four percent. But the lean mass, which includes muscle and bone, didn't see any changes at all.

In addition, there were big improvements that were seen in the LDL (low-density lipoprotein) and triglyceride levels. The growth hormone increased, which was important in helping the participants maintain their muscle mass. To take this even further, some studies show that eating just one meal each day resulted in a significant amount of fat loss, even if that meal included the same number of calories as eating three or more times during the day. The most important thing here, though, is that there was no evidence of muscle loss at all.

Let's take this even further. More recently, a randomized trial of fasting versus caloric restriction found that there really wasn't any evidence that muscle was burned up during the fasting process. During this same trial, the fasting group was told to follow the 36-hour fasting protocol every other day, also known as alternate day fasting. This shows great promise for those who want to get started on fasting for all of the health benefits, but who were scared about the loss in muscle that may result.

According to some experts who seem not to look at the studies above, fasting will burn off 1/3 of a pound of muscle each day that you are on it. What this results in is about 1 pound of muscle a week if you go on an alternate-day fast. This also means that you would see a reduction of 32 pounds of muscle in a group that does fasting for 32 weeks.

However, the actual amount that the fasting group lost over 32 weeks was about 2.6 pounds or 1.2 kg. Yes, this was a little bit of muscle weight loss, but when it was compared to the participants who just went on a calorie restriction, it was less. Those participants who simply restricted their calories ended up losing 16 kg during that same period.

It makes sense that a bit of lean mass is going to be lost when you lose weight. You are losing some of the extra skin and connective tissue at the same time, but the lean mass percentage actually does increase by about 22 percent when you are on a fast.

As you can see, fasting does not burn off a ton of muscle mass, and it won't make you a weak person who is going to suffer from metabolism issues for the rest of your life because you no longer have any muscle mass to deal with. And if you are worried about the slight amount of muscle mass that is lost (which is still less than what you would see with just going on a calorie restriction), then consider adding in some strength training or weight training to your routine to help.

You Can't Exercise When You Are on a Fast

Another misconception is the idea that you are not allowed to work out when fasting. While it is true that you may have to go through and make some adjustments to the way that your workout compared to your normal routine, this doesn't mean that you aren't allowed to work out at all.

When you go on a fast, you are working to deplete the stores of glycogen that are in the body so that you start relying more on the stored fat. During this process, the body may feel a little bit tired and worn down. It is so used to getting the glycogen on a regular basis, and that is a much easier source of fuel for it to rely on than the stored fat. The body will feel weak and worn down for a few days, and sometimes even later on as it adjusts to the fasting regimen.

Because of this, you may need to make some changes to the way that you exercise. Doing the workout right at the beginning of the fast can help because it ensures that you still have some glucose floating around the body to give you energy. Switching to something like HIIT training or weight lifting can be a nice way to ensure that you are still getting a good workout, that you are working on building and maintaining those strong muscles, and that you see even better results from both the fast and autophagy.

Autophagy Means We Have to Overstress Our Bodies

When it comes to autophagy, it is true that the body needs to undergo some stress to make the process happen. This is critical to assuring that the body will start to break down the old parts and build up new ones. If there is no breaking down, then how will there be room for the new cells and parts that you need?

This doesn't mean that we have to overstress our bodies and go crazy. Doing workouts that last six or seven hours each day and are incredibly intense, or fasting for a month straight may seem like they will help out more, but you will find that there are actually more effective, and easier, methods for starting the body on this process.

Simple exercise, such as an intense 30-minute workout or HIIT training, can be enough to help when you are looking to enter into autophagy. Going on a fast that is a few days long, or even just a one-day fast, can be enough to get the body started with autophagy. And these are much easier to start and maintain compared to the more intense options above. Autophagy needs a bit of stress to get started, but that doesn't mean that you have to go crazy in order to see the results.

Autophagy can be a great process for your whole body. It ensures that the body can function properly because it gets all of those old cells and proteins and other parts, and removes them so that new ones can start. It is a simple concept to work with, but you will find that it really does make a difference throughout your whole body.

Chapter 4: Two Ways to Water Fast

Now that we have spent a bit of time talking about the benefits of fasting, it is now time to look at the different methods of fasting that you have available at your disposal. There are two main types of fasting: intermittent and extended.

When we talk about intermittent fasting, we are usually talking about fasts that will last for about 24 hours or less – though sometimes they will go for a little bit longer. These are short fasts that you can implement into your daily routine and still provide you the benefits of autophagy that you are looking for, without having as big of a challenge.

When we are talking about extended fasting, it usually means a fast that lasts between seven to ten days. These fasts may pose more of a challenge since you are going without food and any calories for at least seven days. However, the benefits that you can get out of these fasts are amazing and can really ensure that autophagy has the time it needs to be successful.

Let's take a closer look at the way that these two fasting styles work so that you can decide which one is the best for you!

What Is Intermittent Fasting?

Intermittent fasting has become very popular as a way to help manage calories and lose weight, without all of the counting and other concerns that come with a traditional dieting plan. There are also many different protocols that come with it, which makes it easier for individuals to get on the fast and find the one that works the best for them.

When it comes to intermittent fasting, you are going to learn how to extend out the periods of not eating during the day, and limit how much time you are allowed to eat from one day to the next. It really is as simple as that. As long as you are careful about the foods that you are eating and you stick with your periods for eating, you will find that it is easier than ever to get weight loss and health benefits with intermittent fasting.

There are a variety of different methods that you can choose to go with when it comes to starting your own intermittent fast. The most common method is the 16/8 method. For this, you will limit your eating window to just eight hours a day, and then the rest of the day you rely on water and other non-caloric beverages to keep you hydrated. This is as simple as finishing your evening meal and not having any late-night snacks and then skipping breakfast the next day. Different variations come with this method, but they all basically change up how many hours you are allowed to eat and how many you should fast for. The goal is to make the fasting window bigger than the eating window.

Another method that is similar to the 16/8 fast is the warrior diet. For this, you will basically just have water and other non-caloric beverages for twenty hours of the week. You are allowed to have small amounts of fruits and vegetables during that fasting period, but try to keep these under 200 calories as a total. For the final four hours, you can eat one or two bigger meals to help you get the nutrition that the body needs to stay healthy.

The warrior diet can be hard to go on, especially since it is a fasting regimen that is supposed to happen every day of the week. Many people start out with some of the smaller fasting lengths and then build up to this, or just implement this period into their routine on occasion. You can mix and match to find the method that seems to work the best for you.

The 5:2 diet is another option that works well with intermittent fasting. When you go on this version, you will pick two days that you will fast on. These can be any two days of the week, as long as they are not right next to each other. So going on a fast on Tuesday and Thursday is fine under this kind of protocol. During those two days, you need to keep your calories at no more than 500 for women and 600 for men. You can choose how you would like to divide up the calories based on your own needs. Some people will split these calories into two different meals, and some like to wait until the end of the day and have all of the calories at the same time to help them not go to bed hungry. For the other five days of the week, you are required to eat a diet that is healthy and full of nutrition to help the body out.

Alternate day fasting is a popular method as well. For this one, you will go on a fast every other day. Some protocols ask you to go on a complete water fast, and others are fine if you choose to add in up to 500 calories. These can sometimes be turned into a 36-hour fast pretty easily as well. You should decide whether you are going to add in the calories or not, and then do some meal planning because this kind of fasting method can be intense.

The eat stop eat method is a nice one to choose as well. For this, you are going to get on a 24-hour fast. You will eat normally one day, stop eating for 24 hours, and then go back to eating normally. This one doesn't have to be as hard as it sounds. Simply stop eating after dinner one night, and then wait until dinner the next day before you eat again. This would give you a 24-hour fast and all of the benefits that come with it.

There is also the crescendo fasting that we talked about in a previous chapter. This is a good way for you to adjust your eating habits and get used to the new eating plan. You may find that intermittent fasting is quite a bit different than the eating plan that you are currently on. Many Americans are going to spend almost every waking moment eating. They start their day off with some breakfast, eat at lunch and dinner, and have a few snacks along the way. Going from eating all of this down to a more restricted eating window can be tough for anyone. The crescendo fasting, as well as other options, will help you deal with this by having you just fast a few times a week for shorter periods so that you can build up to some of the other fasting types.

There is not necessarily an eating plan that comes with intermittent fasting. You are allowed to eat whatever diet you would like when you are out of your fasting times. The thing here is that if you are not careful with the foods that you consume, then you will still end up gaining weight and not see the results that you want, even if you do go on this kind of fast.

As long as you eat meals that are healthy and full of nutrition, you are going to be amazed at the results that you can get with intermittent fasting. If you are looking for a method that seems to work really well, and many people are combining with their fasts, then you may want to go with the ketogenic diet as your eating plan.

The ketogenic diet is a low carb, high fat, moderate protein diet plan. It can help you to feel full and satisfied, which makes the fasting times easier to handle. In addition, it forces the body to enter into the process of ketosis faster than before, intensifying the results that you are trying to get when you go on a fast.

All of the methods of intermittent fasting can be very effective. Some of the methods that may be considered a bit easier are going to show results a little slower, but then you won't struggle on them as much. Some of the other methods that may pose more of a challenge, such as alternate day fasting, will provide you with the benefits even faster.

Make sure that you thoroughly research the fasting method that you want to go on before you get going. Each of the protocols will ask for slightly different rules, and it is important that you know the rules that go with your chosen fast. The good news is that these protocols, even though they go on a shorter fasting window than the extended fasts, can still show you many great health benefits over time, and they are easier to maintain over the long term.

Many people have decided that intermittent fasting is the right option for them. First, they can get many of the same benefits from going on an intermittent fast as they can with the extended fasts, plus these smaller fasts are often going to be much easier to handle. If you only have to do a few hours of fasting on a daily basis, or one or two all day fasts a week, it is much easier to handle than trying to go on a fast for a week or longer.

There are also many different options when it comes to starting an intermittent fast. You can choose which protocol you like the best, and you will get results from it. Some protocols are easier than others, which makes them perfect for any level of faster you are. If you are a beginner and a little nervous about getting started, then you can always start with a smaller daily fast and build up as you want. If you have done dieting for some time, or you need to heal some serious health conditions quickly, then you may want to consider going on one of the tougher fasts, such as the 5:2 or the alternate day fast.

Adding intermittent fasting into your day can be really easy. You may even pick out a certain protocol based on what works best for your schedule. And you don't have to worry about taking time off from work to rest because most of these fasts aren't going to wear you out as much as the extended fast will do. So, if you have one or two days at work that are really busy and you barely have time to eat on those days anyway, consider doing the 5:2 method and not eating until the end of the day for your 500 calories. If you barely have time to eat breakfast, consider going on the 16/8 fast plan and stop eating after supper and don't have breakfast in the morning.

It is super easy to start on an intermittent fast, and there are a ton of options out there to help you get in the best health and feel amazing. You just have to decide which method you want to go with and then get started!

What Is Extended Fasting?

Another form of fasting that you may want to try out is an extended fast. While intermittent fasting usually doesn't go much above 36 hours in most cases, although there are times when it may go up to 72 hours, an extended fast is going to work to make you fast for a longer period. Most of the extended water fasts will go somewhere between seven and ten days depending on the goals of the person following it and the amount of willpower and determination that they have. In some cases, the extended fast may last for fourteen days or a little longer, but these lengths are usually done under the supervision of a medical professional.

Fasting can provide the individual with clarity, increase how productive they are, and even extend their lifespan if used properly. Two main benefits come with fasting, and both of them can help your body heal itself and function much better than before. The first benefit is autophagy, which we have discussed in-depth in this guidebook and is the process that occurs naturally in the body where old cells are recycled, and new ones are created. The second main benefit of fasting is ketosis, which is when the body starts to use its own natural fat stores to help keep you energized.

Going somewhere between seven to ten days without any food and only enjoying water may seem a bit crazy, but this is the practice that is known as extended fasting, and it has become very popular. It is a method that will help you to challenge yourself a bit, but the rewards and the payoff are definitely worth all of the hard work. There are even a bunch of different gadgets and other pieces of technology that you can try out to track your different vital signs and make sure that you are doing well.

Extended fasting is going to be a bit different than intermittent fasting, but it can provide you with many of the same benefits that you are used to if you ever went on that kind of fast. Because of intermittent fasting, many different protocols have come up that are considered fasts. You can go on one that has you fast a few days a week, as long as you don't do those days consecutively. Some will have you not eat anything after supper and then not eat breakfast the next day. Research has shown that for at least some people, some great health benefits can come for most individuals who follow these kinds of eating patterns.

However, extended fasting is a bit different. Technically, extended fasting is going to be any fast that goes for more than 24 hours, but since some of the intermittent fasting protocols fall into this kind of category, it has been expanded to cover a fast that usually lasts a week to ten days. This kind of fasting works similarly and is going to provide you with some of the same benefits as your intermittent fasting – but it does belong to a different category because it is considered much more extreme compared to the other methods of fasting we have discussed.

Instead of missing out on a meal here or there, extended fasting takes away your solids for up to a week. Many people choose to go on an extended fast to help them lose weight, but this may not be the goal for everyone. Some people like the amount of mental clarity they can get when they go on an extended fast – and others want a quick fix to help them deal with some of their major health concerns.

If you are looking to lose weight, improve your concentration and focus, and help yourself reach an optimal level of health, then extended fasting may be the best choice for you. And a water fast during this time can help you feel hydrated and provide you with a ton of great benefits. Many people have gone on an extended water fast to improve their high blood pressure, solve issues with weight, help with insulin sensitivity, and so much more.

It is common to find that many of the individuals who do extended fasting are men, but there is a growing number of women jumping on board for this system as well. There are also different protocols that you can follow with this, and some people decide to build up to it, maybe starting with some of the different methods of intermittent fasting until they can build themselves up to the longer fasts of a week.

There is no denying that any kind of a fast, whether it is for one day, one week, or even longer, can bring about some side effects that are pretty unpleasant, especially for someone who is new to the idea. You are going to feel hungry during this time because your stomach is missing out on food. However, if you can keep yourself hydrated and find ways to distract yourself (as well as relaxing when needed), some of these issues will pass – other common side effects that may come up include headaches, trouble with sleeping, heartburn, irritability, and brain fogs. Even those who do this kind of fasting all the time now will state that this kind of extended fast can be hard until you gain some more familiarity with it.

It is going to be hard to get started with this long of a fast, but if you eat a diet that is healthy, both before and after the fast, you can still provide your body with the nutrients it needs to do well, and you can get all of the benefits of these longer fasts. Once you have done the fasts a few times, you will adjust and find many of the side effects dissipating and not bothering you as much. Just make sure that you take some breaks between your week-long fasts, so you give your body time to stock up on healthy nutrients and give it time to heal from the autophagy.

For your first extended fast, it may be best to stick with a time limit that is between five to seven days. You can always expand out later if you decide that this is the right choice for you. However, if you are not used to fasting, then it can be hard to take on more time than that for the first few opportunities that you get with it.

If you decide that going on an extended water fast is the right option for you, then it is time to get started. For this to work, you need to pick out the day and timeframe that you want to use for the fast. You get some freedom here, but it may be best, at least for the first few fasts, if you chose to just do it on days that you have off, or days that you can take off. You are going to feel a bit tired and worn out when you get started with the fast. While these will fade off after a few days, it is a good idea to give your body some time to rest and relax as it adjusts to the new fasting regimen.

You also need to make sure that you keep plenty of water nearby when you are on one of these longer fasts. Many people forget that even though they are not eating, they still need to take the time to drink plenty of water to keep themselves hydrated. Remember that not only do you need to drink the amount that was required before you went on the fast, but you are also missing out on about twenty percent of your daily water from the foods you usually eat, so add that in as well. Some of the worst side effects happen because you aren't getting hydrated enough, so work on preventing this problem from the beginning.

During this time, make sure that you find ways to distract yourself. Your hunger and lack of food situation will become a whole lot worse if you allow yourself to sit around and only focus on that. Consider finding some books to read, going out with some friends and doing something that is not food related – go on a walk, or binge watch some of your favorite shows. Just make sure that you are busy. You may even find, just like other people who go on an extended fast, that it actually feels pretty good to be up and moving and that you can get more done more productively.

Make sure that you listen to your body during this time. Some people can do the seven days and feel fine, although a bit hungry at the end. However, others may get to day four or day five and start to feel sick. They may not be drinking enough water or dealing with a serious complication. If you feel that something is wrong, make sure you go and visit your doctor right away.

While there are some risks for going on an extended fast, and these risks can be really important to watch out for if you are dealing with certain medical conditions, most people have decided that the payoffs are worth it all. The biggest thing to watch out for, during this kind of fast, is your own medical conditions. And if you are doing this just to lose weight quickly, then the weight is likely to come back. If you are using it as a way to improve your overall health and make you feel amazing, then this can be a great fast to go on.

You also need to be careful of the different health issues that can come up. While fasting can be very good for the body, having many periods where the body isn't getting calories can be hard on the body. For women, in particular, you have to be careful about how it could disrupt your hormones, cause insomnia, cause brain fog, and increase anxiety. Add to this that, in some cases, extended fasting can cause a reduction in fertility, and it is important to take precautions as a woman when going on one of these longer fasts.

For those who have certain medical conditions, or who are just a bit worried about how the fasting works and they want to be extra careful, doing this kind of fast under the supervision of a medical professional may be best. As long as you are not trying to conceive, and aren't nursing or pregnant, these fasts can go very well. In addition, those who are dealing with insulin-dependent diabetes, adrenal fatigue, and thyroid problems can benefit from having a medical professional watch over them as they go through the fasting.

When it comes to promoting the process of autophagy, you will find that both of these methods of fasting can be very effective and provide you with a ton of benefits in the process. Some find that they like going on the extended fasts because they provide the most benefits in a short amount of time, and can make one feel great. For others, they may find that going on a longer fast is just too hard for them to manage, and they can benefit from the shorter bursts of fasting that are prominent with intermittent fasting.

Chapter 5: Important to Note – Things to Consider When You Start Fasting

At this point, you may be ready to jump in and get started with your fasting. There are many benefits, and fasting is one of the best and fastest ways for you to enter into the process of autophagy. You know the benefits, you are excited to see what will happen, and you are ready to get the most out of fasting and all it has to offer.

However, there are a few aspects that you need to consider so that you can get the most out of this kind of eating plan.

Some of the Negative Side Effects

Many great benefits come with fasting, and we have talked about quite a few of them already in this guidebook. However, there are a few side effects that can occur when you first get started with fasting. These are pretty mild, and most of them are going to go away when you are used to fasting for a few weeks. Some of the negative side effects that you need to be aware of when you get started with any type of fasting include:

Hunger and cravings

These may not seem like a big deal, but when you are dealing with the fast and get to the end of it, your hunger and cravings will become crazy and be the only thing that you think about with fasting.

Of course, when you are done with a fast, you are going to feel hungry. You have gone for a long time without eating anything. Your stomach is going to be empty, and the body will want to eat something in order to feel better. The only way to deal with this hunger is to eat something. As soon as the fast is done, you can have a meal, and this side effect will go down. After some time, the body will be able to adjust to the fasting, and you won't feel as hungry. Until that time comes, find ways to distract yourself so that you don't focus on the hunger as much.

You may also notice that you have a lot of intense cravings when it comes to being on a fast. Your body wants to get that glucose back, and so if you are not careful when you are done with the fast, you may give in to these cravings and eat more than usual.

It is fine to give in to those cravings on occasion, especially right after the fast is done. This helps you to satisfy that craving rather than ignoring it and makes you feel less deprived. Just make sure that you work on a meal plan and include that craving into the first meal, rather than just letting your cravings go crazy. This helps you to stay within your calorie recommendations and makes it easier to see the results that you want without going overboard.

Heartburn and bloating

Your stomach is still going to produce a lot of acids, even when you stop eating for a bit, and this acid is so important for helping you digest food. On a traditional diet, you will often eat every few hours or more. This causes the body to get into the habit of producing acid every few hours to handle the food. However, when you go on a fast, those acids are still there, being produced, even though there isn't any food in your stomach to handle it. Because of this, it is common that you may experience heartburn.

This heartburn can range from just a bit of discomfort to burping all day to even full-on pain. Time is going to help with this side effect. As you spend more time fasting, the body will get better at regulating the acid that is produced, and it will go away. Make sure that you drink plenty of water on your fast, prop yourself up a bit when you go to sleep. And then, when it is time to eat after the fast, don't eat spicy or greasy foods that will make the heartburn worse. If this symptom doesn't go away, then it may be time for you to speak to your doctor about it.

Feeling cold

This side effect is noted less often than others, but some people who go on a fast do find they become colder. This could be because the digestive system slows down during this time because there isn't any food for the stomach to digest. As a result, the body won't release as much heat. Make sure to dress warmly and keep some blankets on hand to ensure that you don't feel too cold during this time.

Headaches

Some people who go on a fast get headaches at the beginning, which can be from a lack of food or lack of energy. Sometimes it can even be from not getting enough water and relaxation. If you feel that these headaches are becoming a big issue, you need to sit back and relax more and make sure that you are drinking plenty of water, as hydration is a major cause of headaches.

Low energy

One common complaint that comes up with people who are ready to start on fasting is that they feel low on energy. It is possible that you will feel a bit lethargic and tired when you first go on a fast, and this can make it hard to have any motivation to get anything done. It can also make it harder to stick with the type of fast that you want and ensure that you get results.

There is a good reason for all of this happening. We brought this up a bit before, but basically, the body is used to relying on glucose, from the carbs and sugars that we consume in our diet, for its fuel source. Glucose is really easy to get hold of in your body, and the cells don't have to do a ton of extra work in order to make these into fuel. It may be easy for the body, but glucose is a very inefficient source of fuel.

In many cases, we don't use it all up. We may still be hungry for more because the glucose will be in the bloodstream and not the stomach, but not used up. This extra glucose is then stored in the body as excess fat and can accumulate all around the body. We end up in a vicious cycle of taking on more and more glucose that we don't need, but which the body wants to use as fuel.

When you go on a fast, especially one that is a bit longer, the body has to learn how to rely on something other than glucose for energy. For the first twelve hours, it will rely on the glucose to keep it healthy and strong. However, if your fast lasts for longer than that, the body has to search for another fuel source. This can take some time for the body to do, and in the meantime, you will feel tired and low on energy.

After some time, the body will become more adjusted to going straight to using fat to keep you energized, and the process is not going to take so long. You may find that you have even more energy than usual when this happens. Until that time, make sure that you stay hydrated, and give yourself some time to rest so that you can stick with the fasting and all of the benefits that come with it!

Overeating

After you go on a fast, you are going to be hungry. All of the protocols will have you going longer than usual without eating anything. Going that long can be healthy for you and will provide you with some of the health benefits that we talked about above, but it will still make you feel hungry when everything is done. Because of this, it is very important that you watch out for what you eat when you are done.

As you get to the end of a long fast, you are going to have a lot of hunger and a lot of cravings that you need to deal with. This is completely normal, but if you are not careful, you will easily end up overeating and making yourself uncomfortable. Think about it, yes, you are hungry, but your stomach has been empty for a long time. If you just dive into everything that you see right when the fast is done, this is going to cause a number of problems.

The first problem that can arise is making yourself feel uncomfortably full. You will have trouble stopping yourself from eating too much because when you eat fast, the stomach can't signal to the brain quick enough that it is done. This can make your stomach hurt and be a general discomfort. In addition, when you eat this fast and this much, it is easy to take in too many calories. Part of the benefits of going on a fast is that it can help you to restrict your calorie intake and ensure that you lose weight. If you overeat, that all goes out the window.

It is natural to be hungry when the fast is done, and you will probably want many things that are comfort foods, with lots of sugars and carbs. The best way to handle the end of your fast and to ensure that you don't overeat is to do a meal plan. Before you go on the fast, consider sitting down and planning out your meals. This allows you to figure out what you will eat after the fast, and before the fast, and you can make smarter choices when the fast is done, and you are hungry.

Brain fog

In the beginning, you may feel as if there is a fog around your brain. Brain fog as well, as a general feeling of being sluggish, is pretty common when you get started on a fast as you get used to it all. The good news is that as you adjust to the fast, and you get a chance to let the body find its new source of fuel outside of the regular and easy to find glucose, then the brain fog is going to go away. In fact, some studies that show that going on a fast and implementing it into your life for a long time can improve how well the brain can function.

While there are a few different types of negative side effects that can happen when you go on a fast, whether it is an intermittent fast or an extended fast, most of these are going to be pretty short term. You won't have to worry about them staying around for a long time, and if you can make it through a week or so with these side effects (for the shorter-term fasts), then you will see some amazing results and the side effects will go away.

How Long Should You Go On a Fast?

The next thing to consider is how long of a fast you would like to go on. This can depend on a number of factors. You have to consider what health condition you are dealing with, your previous diet, whether you want to implement this into your health routine, and more.

First, we are going to take a look at the health condition that you are going to solve with the fast. If you just want to improve your overall health, then it is a good idea to go on one of the protocols from intermittent fasting. You can easily add in this kind of fasting on a regular basis, choosing a daily fast, or going on one that is a bit longer one or two times a week and still get the benefits. However, if you have a major health concern that you need to get fixed quickly, and you want to get a head start on it, doing an extended fast that lasts between seven to ten days may be the best bet.

This can be incredibly effective when it comes to things like high blood pressure. Studies have shown that patients with blood pressure that was considered high were able to reduce their pressure drastically in a seven-day fast. Those who had higher blood pressures were able to see even more dramatic changes. These changes can happen with intermittent fasting, but not as quick. For people who have blood pressure readings that are getting out of control, it may be time to consider going on an extended fast to get it under control.

In addition, you need to worry about the seriousness of the health condition that you already have. For some situations, it may not be a good idea to go on a longer fast. This could make the situation worse. That doesn't mean that one of the shorter fasts offered with intermittent fasting may not be the right option for your needs.

The next thing to consider is the diet that you are on before you start the fast. For those who are on a traditional American diet, it may be hard to switch straight from that over to a ten-day fast. The body is used to having a constant supply of food and glucose available to it, and switching off suddenly can be a big challenge, and can bring out more negative side effects. It may be easier for you to start with a one-day fast a few times a week, or a short daily fast, to help you get started.

This doesn't mean that you can't jump into the longer fast, regardless of what your previous diet was like. However, most people find that going from a lifestyle of excess to one that has nothing at all for that long is difficult. Starting out slowly, and then increasing your times for fasting, can make all the difference in how your health is doing.

What If I Have a Severe Medical Condition?

While fasting can be very beneficial to most people and can provide them with a ton of great health benefits, some medical conditions don't do the best when it comes to this kind of fasting method. Depending on the medical conditions that you have, it may be best to either avoid going on fasting altogether, avoid going on some of the extended fasts or at least go on a fast with the help and supervision of your doctor.

The first condition that you need to watch out for is insulin resistance diabetes. While some symptoms of diabetes can be helped with a fast, especially the shorter-term fasts, you may find that it doesn't work well for you to go on an extended fast without supervision from your doctor. You do not want to go that long without eating when your body relies on the nutrients to keep itself going. If you are going to go on a fast to help with your diabetes, start with a shorter-term fast and see how that goes.

Another group that needs to be careful about going on a fast is those who are dealing with thyroid issues. Your thyroid gland can be in charge of many different hormones in the body. And fasting can cause some issues in the hormone levels as well. In some cases, if the fast isn't monitored properly, and the thyroid issue is bad enough, it could cause more harm than good in these individuals.

Those who are pregnant or may become pregnant soon or who are breastfeeding should never go on one of these fasts. Yes, you may miss a few meals if you are pregnant and dealing with morning sickness. However, there shouldn't be any planned fasting time during any of these periods in your life. Women in these conditions need to provide their body with a constant supply of good nutrition, and this just isn't possible when dealing with fasting in any form.

If you are very concerned about how fasting will affect you and your medical condition, outside of just worrying about being hungry and a little uncomfortable, then it is important to talk to your doctor before you get started with the process of fasting. This allows you to have a chance to discuss the fast with your doctor, ask any questions that you have, and make sure you fully understand the protocol that you are choosing before you get started.

Chapter 6: If Fasting Is Not for You – Ways to Achieve Autophagy Without Fasting

We already know that many great benefits come with entering into the autophagic process. This process allows your body to clean up much of the waste that would otherwise hang around, reduce inflammation, prevent a ton of common diseases and aging issues, and help our bodies feel better. The main way that people are going to induce autophagy is with the help of fasting – as we have talked about in the rest of this guidebook.

However, for some people, fasting is not an option. Maybe they have tried it for some time, and they can't keep up with it, so they need to go with something else. Maybe the fasting plans just aren't best based on their medical history. For others, fasting may work, but they want to try something else along with it to get some more pronounced results.

The good news here is that there are different methods that you can follow to help induce the autophagic process. Whether you do these at the same time as a fast, or on their own, they can induce autophagy and help you get all of the great health benefits. Let's take a look at some of the other methods of inducing autophagy that you may want to consider for your health and lifestyle.

Exercising

The typical American spends a lot of time sitting around the house, or at their jobs, or doing other things during the day. They don't get the amount of movement that they should, and they feel worn out and tired all the time. However, another problem that can come when you don't exercise is that you aren't allowing the body time to clean itself out via the natural processes that come with exercising.

It is possible for exercise to be enough to induce autophagy, especially when you do more intense workouts at least a few times a week. This is because, like exercise, autophagy is going to respond to stress on the body, and exercise is going to work by creating a bit of damage to the tissues and muscles. These damages are small and not such a big deal, but they are a natural part of the detoxification process that comes with autophagy.

The small damage that occurs may be natural, but then the body will go in and make repairs to these small damages. This helps to clean out the body and can ensure that you become leaner and stronger in the process. Even smaller spurts of exercise a few times a week may be enough to turn this process on.

In addition, research shows that exercise is going to help increase the amount of blood flow and vasodilation that occurs throughout the body. This increase in blood flow can make us feel better, and it hurries up the cleaning out process.

One study that was done on mice involved giving the animals substances that made their autophagosomes a glowing green color. These are the structures that are going to surround the wastes of the cells or the other parts that the body is going to recycle. It was found that when the rats ran on the treadmill for at least 30 minutes, the amount of glowing green in the mice ended up increasing.

This speed seemed to keep on increasing until the mice reached about 90 minutes of running. This means that the mice were able to demolish their cells just by running and doing some cardio. Exercise can definitely be a quick way for the body to induce autophagy on its own and make you feel great in a short amount of time.

The good news is that it seems any kind of exercise is going to be efficient. You don't have to spend hours on the treadmill just to see a little bit of autophagy happen. Any kind of training that is a bit higher in intensity, and that can get your heart rate up, will help you with this process. You should aim to get about twenty to 30 minutes of this kind of exercise into your day in order to see the autophagic process happen. Getting a little extra on occasion can help as well.

This means that it is time to implement a good and regular exercise program into your daily routine. There are many great exercises out there, and you may find that implementing a few of them into your schedule, and mixing and matching them a bit, can make it easier to stick with the workout plan and ensure that you don't get bored with the experience. Try to aim for a good mixture of flexible and stretching, weight training, and cardio to get the best results.

The Ketogenic Diet for Autophagy

If you are not interested in going on one of the fasts that we have talked about in this guidebook, but you are still interested in getting into the process of autophagy, then following the ketogenic diet may be the answer you are looking for. This is a great diet plan that reduces the amount of glucose that you take in, whether it comes in the form of carbs or sugars, and forces the body into the same fat burning process that you find when you spend time on a fast. However, you can get into that fat burning mode without having to go long periods without eating.

When we look at the ketogenic diet, we notice that it is a very low carb, moderate protein, and high fat kind of diet. This is very much the opposite of what we are used to seeing in a traditional American diet, which is why it is successful for so many people. The idea with this diet plan is that we want to take in as many of our calories from the fats that are found in food, and as few calories from carbs as we can.

First, let's take a look at the fats. It is recommended that you aim for 60 to 75 percent of your daily calories coming from fats. This is a high number and can take some time to adjust to, but it will do wonders for turning your body into a fat burning machine and can help you to stay full and focused. There are a lot of great sources of healthy fats, such as butter, olive oil, and even fats that are found on various meat sources.

Next comes the protein sources. You will want to get about twenty percent of your daily calories from protein. This ensures that you are getting enough protein to keep the muscles strong and lean, especially if you are adding in a workout plan to all of this, but also ensure that the majority of your calories are going to come from the fat we talked about before. There are many great sources of protein that you can go with. You can focus primarily on protein sources that have some heavier amounts of fats as well, but any protein source can work well. Just make sure that you stay away from breaded and fried options because these are going to add in more carbs as compared to what we are allowed on this diet plan.

And finally, we need to focus on keeping our carb content as low as possible. It is recommended that you only keep about five percent of your daily calories set aside for your carb intake. This can sometimes be hard to do, but it ensures that you can enter the process of ketosis. When you are picking out your carbs, don't waste them on things like pasta, desserts, and other baked goods, etc. Instead, make sure that you are getting a wide variety of vegetables, and maybe some fruit, so you can get more nutrition out of the few carbs that you get.

The whole point of limiting the carbs so much on the ketogenic diet is to ensure that your body enters ketosis. With this process, the body can give up its dependence on glucose, and will instead focus on using fats, either the fats that we eat or the fats that are stored in the body, to help keep it energized and doing well. This is a great way to clean out the body and can make the individual feel healthier because they don't have to rely on the glucose any longer.

Some people who are dealing with many different health problems, or those who want to lose weight, may find that it is best for them to go on a combination of a fast and the ketogenic diet. Adding these both together can help the body achieve the autophagic process. With that said, fasting isn't the right option for some people. If this is the case with you, then it may be a good idea to go with the ketogenic diet and see what benefits it can provide your body.

Getting Enough Sleep

Failure to get enough sleep can interfere with the process of autophagy. This is because much of this process is going to occur while we are asleep when we don't have our resources put towards other things.

In one animal study, it was confirmed that sleep deprivation altered the process of autophagy, allowing all of those dead and damaged cells to hang around the body. What this means is that you must make sure that you get enough sleep each night, and ensure that you stay on the same sleeping schedule to see the best results.

In our modern world, it is sometimes hard to get the amount of sleep that we really need as we spend so much time working, going to school, running to activities, trying to meet up with friends, cleaning the house, and trying to get a million other things done during the day. Then, at the end of the day, we are either still doing more work, or get distracted by social media and other things. It isn't uncommon to go many nights without getting the full eight to nine hours of sleep that you need to see the autophagic process in action.

There are a number of things that you can do to ensure you get enough sleep on a day-to-day basis. Some tips include:

• Set a bedtime: And stick with it, even on the weekend and other days off. The closer you can maintain your set bedtime, the better off you will be. It ensures that you can fall asleep at the same time each night, and can make it easier to wake up the next morning. Even if you have a day off or nowhere to be the next day, it is important to stick with the same bed and wake up time.

• Get into a routine: The best thing that you can do when you are trying to get more sleep is to set up a bedtime routine. The point of this is that once the body gets used to the routine, as soon as you get started with the first task, the brain will start gearing up to fall asleep and you won't have to put in as much work as before. The bedtime routine doesn't need to be something that is overly complicated and hard to follow. You could make it as simple as taking a bath, brushing your hair, brushing your teeth, reading a chapter in a book, and then going to bed.

• Turn off your phone and avoid screen time: Screen time can really mess with your sleeping patterns. It is best to turn off your phone, shut down your computer or laptop, and stop watching a movie at least a bit before you are ready to go to bed. This can be so beneficial to the brain and the body and makes falling asleep much easier.

• Spend some time reading: After a long day of work or school or anything else that has gone on, it is often hard to calm right down. You should have a transitory time between all that craziness of the day and the time you go to bed. Spending a few minutes, even just fifteen minutes, reading at the end of the day can help keep you calm and make it easier to fall asleep.

• Turn the lights off: Don't go to bed with the light on. This light can interrupt your sleep and confuse the body. If you must have a light, keep a small nightlight somewhere out of the way.

- Don't turn the television on in your room: One of the worst things that you can do when it comes to your sleeping schedule and how deeply you fall asleep is having a television in your room. Some people swear that this is the only way that they fall asleep, but in reality, it is messing with their REM cycle. Take the television out of your room and replace it with some soothing music instead and see what a difference it makes.

- Keep the room a bit cooler than normal: Most people sleep the best when they have the room at a slightly cooler temperature. You don't have to keep it freezing, but try not to keep it too warm either. You can always cuddle up with an extra blanket to help if needed.

- Get comfortable: It is harder to get to sleep if you find that you feel uncomfortable. Bring in enough pillows, or invest in some new ones, find some sleeping clothes that make you feel good, and bring in blankets. Each person is going to find comfort differently when it comes to their sleeping arrangements, so do what works best for you.

- Silence is best but use nature sounds or classical music if necessary: Silence is often the best way to fall asleep, so you don't feel overwhelmed by the noises that are going on around you. However, for some people, the silence is too hard to fall asleep to. If this is the case for you, then it is fine to turn on some quiet music. Classical music or sounds of nature are the best to lull you to sleep.

Nothing is better than getting enough sleep. It can be hard to see this happen and maintain. However, if you really want to see the results of your efforts, especially if you are working on one of the other options, then make sure you implement a good sleeping schedule into your routine.

Eating the Right Foods

We discussed this a bit when we talked about fasting and going on a ketogenic diet in order to help induce autophagy, but eating a healthy diet is one of the best things that you can do to bring autophagy on in your body. If the body doesn't receive the nutrients it needs to stay healthy, it won't be able to carry out all of the important processes that are needed to keep you going, whether these processes include autophagy or not.

Some of the foods that you should consider adding into your diet to assist with the autophagic process include:

- Turmeric
- Coconut oil
- Green tea
- Coffee
- Ginger

Of course, eating a diet that is well balanced, one that includes many healthy nutrients and minerals, such as what you can get from plenty of fruits and vegetables, is the best way to enter this process. These nutrients are key when it comes time to help the body eliminate waste most effectively.

Protein Fast

This is another type of fasting but is a bit different than the others. You are still allowed to eat, but you will limit the amount of protein that you consume for a short amount of time. You will find that it is possible to get the same benefits that come from autophagy simply by going on a protein fast. For this to work, you will occasionally go on a fast where you eat normally, but you take in 25 fewer grams for the day.

The main idea that comes with this kind of fast is that it allows your body to have a full day to go through and recycle old proteins. These older proteins may not have had a chance to clear themselves out of the body – since they linger around and cause inflammation in the body.

This kind of eating plan will allow the body to clean out all of the cells, without having to worry about muscle loss along the way, helping you to stay lean and fit. These fasts, or lack of protein periods, will only be for a few days so you won't miss out on the protein the body needs too much.

According to one study that has been done on the protein fast, when you can limit the amount of protein that you take in, this will force the body to go through and consume the proteins that are already present in the body – the ones that haven't been used up yet and are becoming toxic in the cells. The way that this eating plan clears out the cells is that it binds the toxins that are found in the cytoplasm of the cell and then moves them out.

Other studies show how being a bit deficient in protein can help to induce the process of autophagy because it is going to work in a manner that is similar to going on a fast, but you won't cut out all of the other nutrients, or go long periods without eating. This is because being deficient in protein reduces both the mTOR and insulin levels, both of which work together to control cell growth and metabolism.

When you can reduce your mTOR levels, and then work to build them back up, it does wonders for helping the body build and repair cells, leading to more lean muscle throughout. This kind of process is also going to help out with controlling aging, as well as preventing disease like diabetes, cancer, and heart disease.

One thing to note is that you don't need to limit the amount of protein that you eat on a daily basis. In fact, having this kind of deficit all the time is going to be a bad thing. You need to have protein in your diet to help build up muscles and to help with many other important processes that occur throughout the body. However, doing this kind of fast on an occasional basis can give the body time to clean up the excess proteins that are found in the cells, allowing it to be more efficient at doing its job.

If you want to go with a protein fast, you will do one that lasts about 24 to 36 hours, just once a week. Some people decide to go with this two times a week and follow the protocol similar to what is found in the 5:2 diet. Remember, you are allowed to eat during a protein fast; you just cut down the grams of protein that you get during that time. The other nutrients can stay about the same.

The protein fast can be a great option to go on to help you enter into autophagy. It promotes a lot of the same benefits and induces autophagy similarly to some of the fasts that we have discussed in this guidebook, without having to spend much time on a long fast and feeling hungry along the way. You may want to give this method a try before starting on a regular fast if you are interested in seeing the benefits of autophagy but have a medical condition that makes it hard to go on a traditional fast.

As you can see, there are several different methods that you can use to induce autophagy. While fasting is often the best and more efficient method and the one that most people will choose to go with first, other methods can prove effective as well. If you are worried about going on a traditional fast, or you are looking for another method that doesn't require you to go hungry, then considering a protein fast, the ketogenic diet, or exercising.

Chapter 7: The Results

If you are looking to get on a fasting regimen or any other diet plan, one of the first things that you need to establish, after determining the rules that go behind it, is the results that you want to achieve. No one wants to spend weeks on a plan, going through times of not eating and working on their willpower only to find out that the real results of that fasting are only two pounds lost over three months.

Often, one of the key parts to find the right motivation you need to stick with a lifestyle change or a diet is having the knowledge and the confidence that it will work. Reading about the success of others when they went on a fast or any other kind of diet and nutrition plan can help you convince yourself that it is possible. You may feel more confident that since they lost the weight, you can as well.

In this chapter, we are going to take a look at some of the various success stories that have shown up concerning fasting – and we've divided them up based on the different protocols that they used to get the results. This helps you to see that fasting really is effective and may be the perfect option for you. It may also help you to choose which of the fasting protocols you like the best if you are stuck on which one to go with.

Linda Christie's Story

Linda Christie was 65 and living in Ashford, Kent when she decided to try out the 5:2 protocol for fasting. In just six months, she lost a total of three stone and dropped from a size sixteen to a size ten. According to Linda, when you get to the age of 60, your health becomes more of a priority. She had the goal of being fit and active for years to come so that she could keep up with her young grandsons, rather than living life as an ailing old lady.

In 2012, she had seen someone talking about intermittent fasting on television. She was intrigued by the promises of health and longevity, and so she decided to give it a try. Before that time, she had weighted about twelve stone and was 5'7". She wasn't what was considered overweight by a lot, but she did know that the extra pounds were impacting her health – she noticed that the weight was painful on her knees, and bending to put her shoes on was a big challenge.

Linda found that the first few days on the 5:2 fast were difficult as she struggled to make it through the fasting days. However, soon she noticed that she was losing around two pounds each week, and that gave her more motivation to carry on. Since she looked after her grandsons a few days a week, she planned her fasting days on the ones when she wasn't looking after them.

For her protocol, she would skip breakfast on these fasting days, then have a bowl of soup for lunch, and then another bowl in the evening with some more vegetables thrown in. Depending on how she felt, she sometimes decided to do a third fast day on Saturday. However, Sunday was always her cheat day of having some donuts at church and maybe a treat at choir rehearsals that evening.

Now that she has reached her goal of getting down to nine stone and four pounds, Linda made some adjustments to her fast and just went on the fast on Tuesdays. That is one of the nice parts of doing this kind of fast. You can make the adjustments that are needed to your daily life, either before or after you reach your goals, to ensure that you maintain it for the long term.

Terri Durrant's Story

Terri Durrant was 56 when she started out with the 5:2 diet. Over the time she tried out this diet plan, she lost about two stone and was able to improve her health. According to Terri, before she went on this diet plan, she was suffering from many different health problems. As a younger woman, she had been a swimmer for Great Britain, but all of that exercise had taken a toll on her body, and as a result, she was suffering from knee and back problems.

At the age of 40, Terri noticed that her weight went up to nearly fourteen stone, and she ended up having to go in and get her knee fully replaced. This meant that Terri was out of action for a long time, which made it very difficult to lose weight, despite trying a few other diet plans. After suffering even more health problems, Terri started out 2014 feeling unhealthy and unfit.

A friend of hers recommended the 5:2 version of fasting, and she decided to go for it, with Tuesdays and Thursdays being her fasting days. Slowly and steadily, the weight started to come off. It took her three months to lose half a stone, but by the time she was on it for six months, she had lost more than a stone. She was able to reduce her clothes size from a sixteen to eighteen down to a twelve to fourteen.

Of course, Terri states that the best part of this fast is that it had such a big impact on her health. She can now keep up with her eight dogs, all of whom are show dogs, and since she is a swim teacher, she has noticed that she is now less likely to catch all the bugs that are going around, including chest problems and bronchitis.

Terri has decided to stick with the two fast days a week for now because she wants to be able to get to the nine stone mark. However, during those fasts, she usually keeps herself to two small meals, one at two pm, and then another when she gets home from work around nine pm. Then, she makes sure that she drinks a ton of water all day. She finds that sticking to a set routine helps her to stay focused and get the best results.

Mimi from Food Can Weight

Mimi is another inspirational story about how well fasting can work to help you lose weight and get in the best health of your life. She found herself at almost 240 pounds by June of 2014 and knew it was time to make some changes to the unhealthy eating patterns that she had developed over the years. She had tried many different diet plans throughout her life and even worked with natural appetite suppressants in the hopes of helping her control her appetite that never seemed to go away. She was even at a point of being scared to lose weight because she feared that losing weight, in the beginning, would only result in her weighing more in the end.

Mimi decided to go through the process slightly differently and focused more on fasting like the Warrior diet. After meeting with some friends who practiced Ramadan, she became curious about the spiritual and health benefits that could come from this. She decided that it might be time to try this out and see how it worked.

She decided to go on a 30-day fast. She was not allowed to have anything during the day except coffee, water, and other beverages without calories in them. Then, at night time before bed, she could eat whatever she wanted. This allowed her to still get in many of the nutrients that her body needed, permitting for a little bit of a splurge, and ensured that she was going to get a lot of fat burning done throughout the day.

By 2016, Mimi had been able to lose 73 pounds in total, bringing her down to just 164 pounds from the almost 240 that she had started at. She noticed that her health felt better, she had a lot more energy, and that this kind of fasting was not as hard to maintain as she had thought. She decided to keep going with this kind of fasting to see how far it could take her.

Zach and the Bulletproof Diet

Zach, a busy business executive, decided to go on the rules of an intermittent fast, but he made it a little bit different. Instead of getting rid of all the calories that were in his diet during the fasting window, he decided to use the bulletproof intermittent fasting method. With this method, a bit of bulletproof coffee in the morning was allowed.

Bulletproof intermittent fasting is very similar to what we see with intermittent fasting, but with the addition of a cup of bulletproof coffee in the morning, rather than eating nothing. The healthy fats that come from the grass-fed butter, along with the Brain Octane Oil, will help you get a good and steady current of energy that will do well for sustaining you through the day. The lower toxins that are found in the beans will help to optimize brain function and the fat loss with high octane caffeine. And the oil will ensure that your metabolism will speed up by twelve percent and increase your ketone production more than ever before.

Of course, if you go on this method, you must make sure that you still eat a healthy diet along the way. The bulletproof coffee can help to keep you full, provides you with energy, and ensures that you are less likely to overeat through the day. However, it is not going to save you if you choose to eat Oreos and Pop Tarts for the rest of the day.

Zach was used to depending on sugar to provide him with the energy needed to get stuff done, and as a result, this resulted in a vicious cycle of him being overweight and miserable. After going on this kind of diet plan, he was able to lose a pound a day for 75 days, without feeling overly hungry all the time.

In addition to losing a lot of fat, Zach noticed that he felt more focused throughout the day, was more alert, and never felt deprived, even though he wasn't eating much. He didn't have to do steroids or other protocols to see the results. He simply had to stop eating at about eight at night, and then, instead of having breakfast, he would have some bulletproof coffee, then wait until lunch to have a meal.

These are just a few of the different success stories that have been found when it comes to intermittent fasting. There are thousands of other stories out there. By going on one of these fasts, or even a longer-term fast, you are getting yourself in the best health possible and ensuring that the process of autophagy occurs for you.

Chapter 8: FAQ About Autophagy and Fasting

As we have discussed, autophagy is the process where the body breaks down old and damaged cells and then removes them. When autophagy is allowed to happen, the cells can use these wastes to stay energized and as fuel to get things done. This is a natural process that should be occurring in our bodies, but thanks to poor eating and diet habits, this process is often delayed or never happens at all.

These broken and damaged parts are completely normal. When you breathe, workout, just live life, and more, the body is going to break down cells and other parts. That is just healthy functioning of your body, which makes room for new parts. The new parts can then do their job, and you feel great with the actions you have to do from one day to the next.

The problem comes when you don't see autophagy occur. Thanks to the unhealthy diets that we have put ourselves on and all of the other toxic environments around us, such as lack of exercise, bad habits, and generally not taking care of ourselves, we have effectively turned off the process of autophagy. Remember, the body needs to go through some kind of stress, such as fast or exercising, in order to enter into this autophagic process. If it never experiences that stress, then it will just keep being turned off and is going to wreak havoc on your body.

With the autophagic process turned off, there is still the issue of broken and damaged proteins and cell parts that are hanging around. These are always going to occur. Even someone who is considered extremely healthy is going to have these wastes produced in the body. It is the way that the body works to repair itself and the way that you get new parts to keep you feeling good and everything working the way that it should.

With a healthy body that promotes autophagy, those wastes are going to be used as fuel and then will pass on through the body. However, when autophagy doesn't occur because the body never goes through one of those good stressors, then the wastes are just going to hang out around the body, and this is never a good thing.

When all of these wastes are left in the body with nowhere to go, it leads to a bunch of problems. First, without a process to go through and clean them up and even to break them down, these wastes are just going to keep hanging out where they were originally put. This prevents new cells and proteins from coming in and doing the job more efficiently for you.

Think of it like having a car. You may look inside and see that some parts are brand-new and some have been on since the car was first made. Just by looking at it, you already know which parts are going to work the best and which ones will struggle. The newer parts will function the most efficiently and will get the job done without any problems. However, the older parts are going to cause problems, can wear on the newer parts, which have to take up some extra work to keep things going, and it won't be long until they break completely.

Simply by replacing these older parts, you can improve the functioning of the car.

The same is true in your body. You need to be able to get rid of all the wastes, so they don't get in the way of the newer parts, and they can even make other parts of the body work harder than usual, causing other parts to get old and worn out at the same time.

In addition, all of these wastes hanging around are known to cause inflammation. This alone can be the root cause of many serious diseases, from high blood pressure to cancer to arthritis, and even more. Autophagy can help solve this issue.

This guidebook has explained many of the methods that you can use to help bring about this autophagic process and to help you get the most out of it once you start. In addition, here are some more things that you need to know before you decide to get started with fasting and to induce the autophagic process.

Do I Really Need Autophagy to Occur?

It is very important that you promote autophagy through the cells. A natural process of the body is to burn out various pieces. These pieces will get old and damaged, just from normal wear and tear from what you do on a daily basis. Autophagy ensures that all of these parts are taken out of the body, without them getting in the way.

Without autophagy, those broken and damaged parts are just going to stick around the body. They will get in the way of new parts forming. The body will continue to use the same old and damaged parts, which is never a good thing for helping you to fight off illness or feel your best. Over time, these broken parts are going to start to cause inflammation and may be the reason that you are suffering from a variety of different diseases, including those related to aging.

Autophagy ensures that this doesn't happen. When older parts are allowed to be removed from the body, it provides newer parts the opportunity to grow and thrive. This helps to give you more energy, makes it easier to lose weight and can prevent a bunch of serious health conditions.

Isn't Fasting Bad for Me?

Many people worry that going on a fast is bad for them. They worry that they are going to harm their bodies and enter into starvation mode. However, it takes a lot more than just a few hours of fasting before you will enter into starvation mode, and it is not going to happen on any of the fasting methods that we talked about in this guidebook – unless you do really bad at following the protocol.

To get into starvation mode, the body has to go a very long time without eating or go a very long time with minimal nutrition. The body has to feel that it is missing out on food and that it needs to preserve what is already has, so it slows down the metabolism. However, if you are going on a fast that is only 24 hours long or less, and you make sure to eat plenty of healthy and nutritious foods during your eating window, then starvation mode is not going to be an issue.

The truth is that fasting has tons of great health benefits that can make you look and feel amazing. Fasting will help you lose weight, get rid of belly fat, lower blood pressure, lower high cholesterol levels, reduce brain fog and other brain problems, and so much more. Even just a short fast on occasion will help you to see great improvements in your overall health, all thanks to the autophagic process.

How Can Fasting Help with Autophagy?

Fasting is one of the best ways to enter into the process of autophagy. Study after study has shown that when the body gets away from using the readily available glucose for energy, it will use the stored fat to keep you going. This process will also instigate the autophagy, which helps to clear out all the toxins and dead and damaged parts of the body that are just getting in the way and causing lots of disease and other issues.

It is best if you can go on a fast that lasts for about sixteen hours. Remember, it takes about twelve hours from your last meal before the fat burning process begins. The sixteen hours ensures that you can spend at least a few hours burning fat, and seeing autophagy occur throughout the body. The longer the fast, the more fat-burning you will see, and the better results you will get.

Can I Enter Autophagy Without Going on a Fast?

Fasting is one of the fastest and most efficient ways to enter into the autophagic process. You only have to go on the fast for a very short amount of time to see this process start up. With that said, there are other options that you can use to help bring about the process of autophagy and help your body get in the best shape possible.

If you are not interested in going on a fast, if you shouldn't go on a fast, or if you are interested in enhancing your fast, then there are a few options available to you. Other ways that you can make sure that you get the most out of the autophagic process include starting the ketogenic diet, eating the right kinds of foods, getting enough sleep, and adding a good exercise routine into your day.

Is There Anyone Who Shouldn't Go on a Fast?

Fasting can be effective for almost anyone who wants to induce the autophagic process and those who want to lose weight and help out a host of other health conditions. However, there are a few people who may find that fasting is not the best option for them.

First, if you are pregnant, breastfeeding, or thinking about getting pregnant in the near future, then fasting is not a good idea. Fasting restricts the nutrients that you take in during the day. While you should be able to make those up during your eating window, you will find that these conditions require you to get a constant stream of nutrition throughout the day. It is better to stay off a fast and wait until after your baby is born, or after you are done breastfeeding.

There are also a number of health concerns that can be aggravated when it comes to fasting. Type 1 diabetes is not always the best for going on one of these fasts, and you may notice that those who have a thyroid condition will often be told not to go on a fast. If you are concerned about how your medical condition will be affected if you decide to go on a fast, make sure to bring up the issue with your doctor.

What Is the Best Length of Fasting for Me?

As we discussed in this guidebook, there are many different fasting protocols that you can choose to go on to help improve your health. As long as you go on a fast for at least twelve hours, although sixteen is usually preferred, you will enter into the autophagic process. Hence, any of the different protocols that we have talked about in this guidebook can work to help you see results.

The protocol that works the best for you may be different compared to what works the best for someone else. If you are hesitant about starting a fast, or worried about how it may aggravate a condition that you already have, then you may want to choose one of the easier daily fasts, such as the 16/8 protocol. On the other hand, if you really want to lose a lot of weight quickly and see your results in next to no time, or you want to help heal a medical condition that has been plaguing you, then going on an alternate day fast or something similar may be a good idea.

Chapter 9: Tips and Tricks to Make Fasting Easier

While there are other methods that you can use to enter the process of autophagy, most people find that going on a fast is the easiest and most efficient method out there. It provides you with quick results, you get many different options to help you out, and it isn't too difficult to follow. With that said, it is a big shift from the way that you ate in the past –and this can be hard for some people to get used to in the beginning.

Fasting is not meant to be a difficult process – it just requires a bit of adjusting and a few tricks to make it work. Some of the best tricks that you can follow to see results when you get started on fasting include:

Start After Dinner

One trick that you may want to try out when you are ready to start with fasting is to make sure that the fast starts after you finish dinner. There are a number of benefits to choosing this as the starting point.

The first benefit is that you won't go to bed hungry. Going to bed hungry is never a positive experience and is one of the main reasons that many people end up failing – or at least really struggling – when it comes to going on a fast. They may have all the ambition to do well, but when they go to bed with their stomachs growling and not being allowed to eat because of the protocol they chose and the amount of time left in their fasting window, they feel miserable.

When you finish the fast after supper, you get the benefit of at least going to bed with a full stomach, and that alone can make the process of fasting so much easier to handle. You will be hungry at some point the next day, but at least you have slept well the night before.

With this method, you will have to skip breakfast the next day. However, the hunger from this can fade pretty quickly. And if you keep yourself busy at work or cleaning the house or getting the kids off to school, etc., you will find that it doesn't take long until you get to lunchtime and you can eat again. This is one of the easiest and most comfortable methods to use to go on a fast, and you will get the best results out of it.

Make Sure That You Drink Plenty of Water

When you go on a fast, or anytime in your life, you should make sure that you drink plenty of water. Water is important for many aspects of your life. It can help you feel hydrated and will keep a bunch of nasty side effects at bay in your body. It can help promote the process of autophagy and makes it easier to dispose of all the waste that is caught up in that process. And water can help to keep your hunger at bay when you are dealing with a fast.

It is very important that you drink a lot of water during your fast. It is easy to become dehydrated during this time, and once you do, many of the negative side effects that we talked about earlier in this guidebook will start to plague you. If you want to limit or reduce these negative side effects, then it is important that you keep a water bottle near you to help keep yourself hydrated.

Make sure that you drink a little bit of extra water than you normally would during the fasting time. Remember, you are not getting your water from food sources during this time, which can mean you are missing up to twenty percent of your liquid content when you are on the fast. Adding in a bit more water to your routine while you do this can really help to keep the dehydration away.

Consider Drinking Some Sparkling Water

This one goes along with the drinking water idea above, but there is a slightly different reason. Yes, it will help to keep you hydrated, and it can be a nice change if you have just been drinking regular water while fasting. For people who are on an extended water fast, plain water is going to get boring pretty quickly, but adding flavoring to the water to make it more interesting will probably throw you off the fast.

However, with sparkling water, you can get a bit of a change to the type of water that you are consuming. That alone can make you feel better and can keep you on the fast for a little bit longer. But another benefit that comes from drinking sparkling water is that it can help keep you full. The bubbles are great for filling up the stomach and making you feel the hunger pains less than before. For those who are going on a longer fast, this can be just the trick you need to make it more manageable to handle.

Coffee Can Help Keep the Hunger Away

Another thing to consider when you need help curbing your appetite is to make sure that you drink a bit of coffee. You don't want to go overboard with this because, for some people, caffeine can cause the jitters and an ill feeling, especially if consumed on an empty stomach. However, having a cup of coffee in the morning while still on your fast can be a great way not only to wake you up but also make some of those hunger cues go away.

If you are going to use coffee to help keep the hunger pains away, make sure that it is black coffee. You can't add sugar and cream or any other additions to the coffee while you are fasting. This may be the way that you liked to drink coffee in the past, but these things are not allowed when you are fasting, and they are going to kick you right out of your fat burning mode. Plus, adding those two things can increase your cravings for the rest of the day if you are not careful.

Find Ways to Distract Yourself

The hardest part of a fast comes when you let yourself sit around and think about food, or think about how long you have until your eating window starts. When you get bored, this will be the only thing you want to think about, and then the cravings and the temptation and the extra hungry stomach will start to take over, and you will feel miserable. When all three of these things start to gang up on you, it is just a matter of time before you cave and go off your fasting protocol.

Instead of letting this happen, make sure that you get out of the house, or at least find other ways to distract yourself. The more that you can concentrate on getting something else done, the less time and energy you have to focus on the fact that you haven't eaten in a bit.

There are many different ways that you can work to distract yourself from hunger pains. Consider making your fasting days the ones that you work most on. You can then sit and work diligently on all projects and other tasks that you need to get done, without worrying about when it is time to eat. In fact, many people claim that they are more focused and more productive when they are on a fast, so this can help you to really speed through the work and get a lot done.

If one of your fasting days happens to occur over a weekend or another day when you aren't at work, then it may be best to consider finding other ways to distract yourself. This can be especially important for some of those longer-term fasts as well. Cleaning the house, working on that one big project that needs to get done, reading, going on a walk, and more can really help you to focus on something other than your hungry stomach.

Finish Your Work in the Morning Before the Fast Is Over, and You Can Eat

Exercise is a very important part of fasting and making sure that you get the results that you want. It can help you burn through the glucose faster, so your body starts to rely on fat burning more. It helps you to feel better and tone the body. It can help you to keep your muscle tone going. And all the benefits of fasting can be magnified when you add in the exercise.

One method that has been pretty successful with exercising and fasting is to get the workout in right at the end of the fast. During this time, you have depleted the extra glucose that has been hanging around the body, and you have, hopefully, been in fat-burning mode for at least a few hours. When you enter into a workout, the body is going to still rely on the fat, intensifying the fat burning results that you can get.

Then, when the workout is done, you can help replenish the body by breaking your fast and having something to eat. This ensures that you get some extra fat burning results while still providing the body with the nutrients it needs after a hard workout. Just make sure that you plan out the meal a bit to avoid overeating on the things you crave, and to help you give your body the nutrients it needs.

Of course, working out at any time of day is very beneficial, so if you find that waiting until the end of the fast is too hard, or you just don't have the time during that period of the day, then it isn't such a big deal. Some people like to work out during their eating window, so they have the nutrients to keep them going on a more intense workout. Some people like to go right at the start of the fast to help push them into fat burning faster. Pick the workout schedule that works the best for you.

Don't Let Others Know That You Are Fasting

It is often best to not let others know that you are on a fast. First off, this gives many negative impressions, and many people may worry that you are doing something to harm yourself. They may not understand why you are doing this, and many may think it is foolish and will try to talk you out of it – but you have personal reasons for going on this fast, and holding on tight to those will make the whole process much easier to deal with.

Telling others that you are going on a fast can be misconstrued as "showing off" and can sometimes set you up for failure. Don't look towards others for the motivation that you need to succeed; instead, look inward and see if you can find your own motivation. What is the main reason why you want to go through all of this? What are you hoping to get out of the process? If you can answer these questions, then you are ready to get started.

Get Out of the House and Away from the Food

Nothing makes fasting harder than just sitting around the house, waiting for your fasting window to be over and your eating window to begin. You are not only going to be bored when you do this, but you are also in close proximity to food during this time. And it is likely that you are going to keep thinking about that food until you get some. How long do you think your endurance and willpower will be able to hold out as you get hungrier and hungrier during the day?

It is fine to stay around the house as long as you have something to do during that time. If you have a big project to work on, some business work to complete, or you even plan to spend the day cleaning, then that is fine. However, if you find that you are just sitting on the sofa watching television, or wandering around aimlessly, hoping that you find some way to bust the boredom and not give in to the hunger or cravings, then this is a recipe for disaster.

When the latter starts to happen, it is time to get out of the house. Even if you just go on a walk for a bit, it is better than being bored in the house where you are likely to make poor decisions and eat foods that you shouldn't. Find some errands to run, meet up with a friend, or head to the library and check out some books – anything that helps you not to sit around and be tempted by food!

Have Some Splurges on Occasion

No one wants to feel like they are deprived all the time. Yes, to see the autophagic process and to lose weight, there are going to be some sacrifices along the way. However, if you are never allowed to splurge and have some fun, then you are going to get bored, and even angry, at your fasting regimen. It is perfectly fine to have a splurge on occasion. It is fine to go out with some friends and push your eating window back a bit. It is fine to eat a few too many calories occasionally. While you should try to keep these down to a minimum, they are not the end of the world.

Don't Feel Bad If You Mess Up Sometimes

As with any kind of diet and eating plan, there are times when you will make mistakes and run into trouble. Maybe you were doing really well on the fast and then, all of a sudden, you ran into trouble and gave in and ate breakfast too soon. This can be disheartening, but again, is not the end of the world.

So what if you didn't make it completely through the fast. You tried hard, and if you followed the protocol well the night before, you still went on a fast for a good amount of time, and you will still get all of the benefits that come with it. Just make sure to plan the rest of your day accordingly. Beating yourself up about this is just going to make the situation worse, and will make it more likely that you will give up and never see any results.

Fasting is one of the best ways to encourage the autophagic process, and it can provide you with a bunch of benefits in the process. However, sometimes, it is hard to make such big adjustments to the way that we eat in order to see these benefits. Following some of the tips that are found in this chapter can make the process much easier to handle overall.

Conclusion

Thank you for making it through to the end of *Autophagy: Unlock the Secrets of Weight Loss, Anti-Aging, and Healing with Intermittent and Extended Water Fasting.*

This guidebook should have been informative and provided you with all of the tools you need to achieve your goals – whatever they may be.

The next step is to take some time to determine which method of inducing autophagy is right for you.

Finally, if you found this book useful in any way, a review on Amazon is always appreciated!

Check out another book by Elizabeth Moore

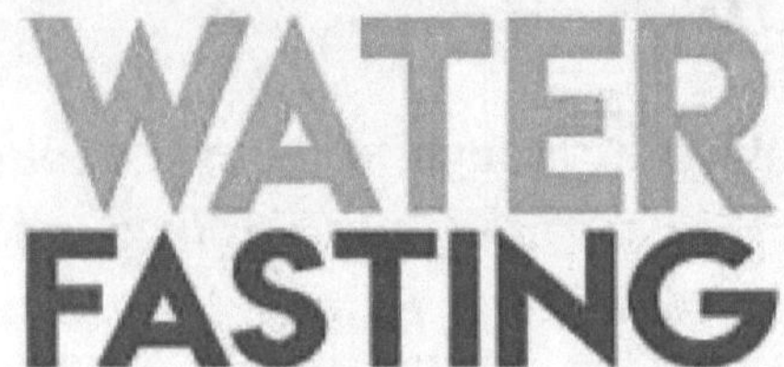

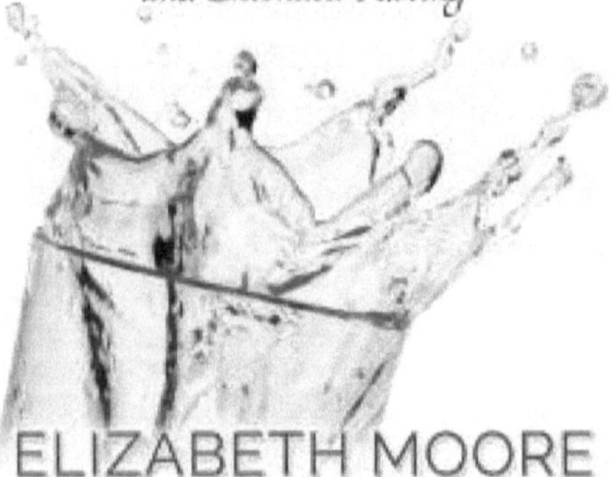

And another one…

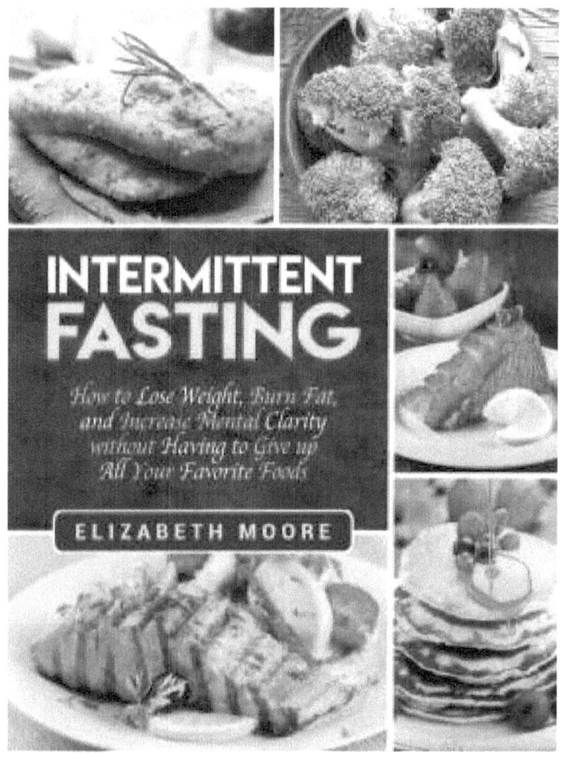